WITHOUT PRESCRIPTION

A GUIDE TO THE SELECTION
AND USE OF MEDICINES
YOU CAN GET OVER-THE-COUNTER
WITHOUT PRESCRIPTION,
FOR SAFE SELF-MEDICATION

by

ERWIN DI CYAN, Ph.D.

LAWRENCE HESSMAN, M.D.

Foreword by

WALTER C. ALVAREZ, M.D.

Simon and Schuster : New York

Published by Simon and Schuster
Rockefeller Center, 630 Fifth Avenue
New York, New York 10020

First printing
SBN 671-21137-4
Library of Congress Catalog Card Number: 77-171603
Designed by Irving Perkins
Manufactured in the United States of America
By American Book-Stratford Press, Inc., New York, N.Y.

CONTENTS

ACKNOWLEDGMENTS

Authors are fortunately not always alone in their endeavors. They depend on cooperation and help in order to complete a task they set out to do.

To see the packages that consumers actually receive, I visited many drugstores to examine the packages and to read their labels. This enabled me also to determine which products were broadly available. Therefore, my thanks go to a number of managers of drugstores in New York, Washington, D.C., and Chicago, who allowed me to examine the products on their shelves. Special thanks are due to Nemiroff Pharmacy in New York for being particularly cooperative.

My secretary, Charlotte Brodkin, deserves thanks for bearing up under drafts, changes, and revisions each time I thought that a better idea struck me.

But I am particularly thankful to Mr. Peter Schwed, publisher of Simon and Schuster, for his personal attention, advice, and guidance. When a quandary on the organization of the book plagued me, Peter Schwed grasped the problem and had an idea toward resolving it. As to the text, it was a mutual endeavor between Dr. Lawrence Hessman and myself, and I am indeed grateful to him.

This acknowledgment would be incomplete without thanks to Professor Philip Miele, who was so vigorous in his assurance of the need for this book and who provided so much intellectual stimulation during its production.

E. D.

FOREWORD

There are on the market many hundreds of nonprescription drugs available, but in a confusing array, so that persons wanting relief from their discomforts do not know just where to turn.

Dr. Erwin Di Cyan, drug consultant to pharmaceutical companies, advising them on pharmacological and other matters pertaining to drugs, has written this book which he hopes will end some of the confusion and help people to decide which of several available nonprescription medicines they may try for relief. A great value of the book is that it can help many a reader to choose which one of two or three available remedies would best serve his needs. Dr. Di Cyan has written as an unbiased adviser, to persons wanting to know more about over-the-counter drugs, and is not writing for any industrial sponsor.

I have known Dr. Di Cyan both as a friend and as an expert drug consultant for some twenty years—he is the man to write this book with integrity, kindliness, and great knowledge of medicine.

WALTER C. ALVAREZ, M.D.

Chicago, Illinois

IMPORTANT!

Be sure to read the Introduction and the other material that follows it in the front of this book before turning to any specific topic and trying to make use of its information. Additionally, each topic has a "Discussion and Cautions" section which *must* be read in conjunction with the subject. Also, the reader is urged to familiarize himself with the possible side effects of certain drugs by consulting the chapter beginning at page 225 and also Appendix B beginning at page 301.

In other words, do not rely upon a separate piece of information about a drug that interests you without making yourself aware of possible accompanying cautionary matters.

NOTE: As this book goes to press, it appears that the FDA will demand that products containing hexachlorophene not be used over the whole bodies of infants, and possibly the order will encompass even more than that. Since hexachlorophene is a component of many preparations, the reader should be aware of the FDA's position.

INTRODUCTION

The purpose of this book is to enable the layman to make an informed choice of the drug products that are available over-the-counter without prescription.

These are known as proprietary or over-the-counter drugs. (Those that are available only on prescription are called "legend drugs," referring to the prescription legend they bear on their label—namely, "Federal law prohibits dispensing without prescription.")

How many times have you been beset by doubts as to which drug product to use for a simple ill, whether it is for acne, indigestion, athlete's foot, or whatever? Have you wondered which advertisement to believe, or what is equally important, *how to interpret it?* If you are a layman you may be stuck: your information comes from biased sources, namely, advertisements, or if it is unbiased, it may come from hearsay on which only dubious dependence can be put.

It is easy to say "don't-use-anything-because-it's-all-no-good." The current vogue to condemn, to deprecate, to debunk most things is a broad philosophy, applied to many facets of our current scene. In large measure it is based on emotion, rather than on the result of thoughtful reflection.

Nonetheless, a problem remains: when you need, say, an antacid or cough mixture, it may be well to have a guide that attempts to answer your questions, rather than to give you the current party line, "it's-all-no-good." Something constructive may answer your questions or your needs. That is our aim in this book.

This book aims to give you an unbiased picture of over-the-counter drugs, particularly what ingredients may be better than others, and it will explain *why* we believe it is so. People buy these drugs for an immediate purpose or to put them into their medicine chest for future use. They should be informed where their best interests lie. Yet, this book is not intended to replace your medical adviser, your doctor.

Often the layman, except in acute or dire conditions, does not really know when a doctor is needed. He is not in a position to exercise judgment in this area. Therefore, if the condition for which you are buying an over-the-counter medicine does persist, see your doctor. Or if symptoms change, see your doctor; any one or more of a dozen developments may be at the root of it.

But if you have to choose in buying a proprietary drug available at your pharmacy without a prescription, use this book to guide you. In order to keep this book to a manageable size—to prevent it from flourishing into a large volume, in which event it would be difficult to use—we have reduced our discussions and have limited our listings to reputable, branded products which are readily and nationally available. Nor did we choose to waste time and space in picking up cudgels to do battle with questionable products—we merely ignored them. But it should not at all be concluded that a product not listed is *ipso facto* no good, nor is a listed product necessarily recommended.

We are thoroughly aware that the claims made in behalf of many over-the-counter drugs have been unconscionably exaggerated. Some just do not do what they promise to do. In our discussion, we base ourselves on their ingredients—the active ingredients are listed on the label—and their virtues and their drawbacks. In some conditions, as obesity, we believe that you should not use any drug.

The fact that we list numerous over-the-counter products available without prescription—and even express a preference for some—should *not* be taken as a recommendation, or even to mean that such products can be, should be, or are usually prescribed by physicians. They are not. Conditions for which patients visit a physician commonly require additional measures, including other drugs, for efficient treatment. Thus the data and products listed here are meant only as a guide, to help an individual to understand better the drugs he would buy anyway over-the-counter without a prescription, for his simple discomforts.

Why do we go to the trouble of frequently listing a long chemical name with 12 to 20 syllables when we also give a shorter name of 3 or 4 syllables? Merely so that the reader has a basis for comparing–is the long name window dressing, label dressing, or an informational designation? There is also another reason: sometimes a short name is a trademarked name, as Duponol C, and the property of the manufacturer. Other manufacturers may often use the same ingredient–which is sodium lauryl sulfate–but cannot use the trademarked name, owned by another firm.

We have been asked by some colleagues who saw the manuscript why we do not give our own formula when we consider it good or superior, rather than list a proprietary product which often costs more. The question is a sound one. But the premise that giving a formula is presumably better than listing an over-the-counter drug is not correct.

If you carry a formula to the pharmacist and ask him to make the product, you may meet certain drawbacks. Here are some:

1. He may not have the material in stock–for example, he may never have heard of attapulgite, which has happened to one of us. We mark a given antidiarrheal as superior because it contains attapulgite–and we give you the reason for it.
2. Proprietary eye drops, for example, are quite high in cost, as compared to the ingredients they contain. But proprietary eye drops are all sterile–a Food and Drug Administration requirement. Most drugstores do not have sterilization equipment to make sterile eye drops.
3. For certain proprietary products–cough mixture, suntan lotion, antacid, etc.–if a pharmacist were to make them

> from a formula that you bring him, they would probably cost more. The reason is sensible: the pharmacist must charge for his time, and that would almost certainly amount to more than the difference in cost between the finished proprietary product and the ingredients of a formula that a pharmacist must compound.

The products listed herein are usually those which are obtainable throughout the United States. The reason for this choice was deliberate: there is little to be gained by our naming a preparation that may have a slight or moderate superiority, but is available only in Washington or, say, a special drugstore in New York or Chicago.

Under the heading of *Ingredients* found in each chapter dealing with a topic, you will find an evaluation of the customary ingredients used in various products. If you refer to that section, you will have a broad view of what certain ingredients do, and why they are included.

Hence, if you are obliged to buy a locally available brand, or prefer to do so on the basis of price, etc., you will be in a better position to judge which product can best serve your purposes.

Moreover, there is an incestuous relationship among the various manufacturers—even among the national distributors, the very large firms. No sooner does a product catch the public fancy—by advertisement or for other reasons—than it is boldly copied by large and respectable and other firms as well. At times even the color scheme is so similar that products resemble each other very closely. There is another reason for closeness of formula: if a copied product departs substantially from the item which it resembles, it may have to meet too many FDA requirements.

Generics: You hear a good deal about generics—and you may hear a good deal more. Is there a difference between generic drugs and trademarked items? (A generic name is one which is in the public domain and which anyone can use since no proprietary rights are connected with it. This differs from a trade name which can be used legally only by the owner of the trade name. For example, petroleum jelly is a generic name, Vaseline a trade name.)

There should not be. Often the manufacturer of a well-known trademarked product is a moderate-to-large firm, and has a tremendous investment in quality control. But with smaller firms who make generic drugs, more often it is not true. These are the facts.

Now, to interpret these facts: the moderate-to-large firms are more vulnerable because they have more to lose. As a matter of self-protection, their testing procedures, which are a large part of quality control, have to be considerably more extensive.

But the gap is becoming narrower. The rigid demands of the FDA's Current Good Manufacturing Practices regulations require the same care from every manufacturer. The gap still exists because the larger or more reputable firm usually exceeds the FDA's demands—for self-protection and perhaps to justify the higher prices that its products cost.

What is more, one cannot deny the fact that new developments—antibiotics and other modern medications—have almost always originated with one of the larger, reputable firms. The manufacturers of generically named drugs have often feasted on the fruits brought in by others.

Nonetheless, many generic products are as reliable as those of the larger, reputable firms. But really it is not possible to answer precisely the general question of whether generics are every-bit-as-good as drugs of established manufacturers.

ERWIN DI CYAN, PH.D.
LAWRENCE HESSMAN, M.D.

May 1971

NOTE

In February 1971, the Food and Drug Administration (FDA) published a proposal which, if promulgated, would in effect remove from the market a great many over-the-counter products that consist of two or more ingredients. Those products are called combinations or combination products.

That proposal would remove from the market those combinations for which the manufacturer cannot offer clinical studies that, by and large, point out that each ingredient of the combination adds to the total effect of the product beyond the mere additive value.

The combination of some drugs is indeed purposeless. Note the types of cough mixtures available 10 to 15 years ago; the combinations—white pine, bloodroot, etc.—were pointless. However, these products have been virtually taken off the market by their manufacturers. It was a matter of commercial attrition; the newer combinations cost appreciably more but are more effective.

To benefit from the effect of a combination is one thing. To be able to prove it—by the refinement of objective methods—is another. And there are not enough clinicians available in the United States, or in any other country, to be able to do those studies.

It would be deplorable to be deprived of combination drugs for simple discomforts. The FDA has been virtually pressured into these steps by congressional criticism. Some border on the ludicrous. It is bizarre indeed that scientists are trained to the bursting point while lay congressmen make the laws.

Under the current demands of the FDA, it would be difficult to justify the existence of such a simple combination as, for example, aspirin-phenacetin-caffeine (APC) tablets.

The original objective of the drug investigations was to inquire why drug prices were so high. Despite that, they have since risen with almost every firm—and risen considerably. The demands on combination drugs, requiring clinical expertise, will probably send the prices of drugs skyrocketing.

Fortunately, in mid-1971 the FDA expressed a less rigid attitude on combinations. Under heavy pressure from physicians and the pharmaceutical industry, the FDA denied that it intended to ban fixed-dosage combinations across-the-board. It even claimed that there are advantages to some combinations, such as patients' convenience and reduced cost. In fact, through its commissioner, the FDA even expressed the view that less stringent efficacy documentation would be applied to over-the-counter drugs.

Unquestionably, private greed is almost limitless—and must be controlled. But perhaps we can learn what happens when government projects itself into a private picture by what took place in Sweden. When Sweden nationalized its drugstores a few years ago, the retail prices of pharmaceuticals increased approximately 25% in the space of about one year.

HOW BEST TO USE THIS BOOK

The table of contents offers a bird's-eye view of the conditions and symptoms described in this book and the classes of drugs used in self-medication for the amelioration of discomforts. Reference first to the table of contents is recommended. However, if retrieval is desired of some specific bit of information previously seen in this book and now sought anew, the index may best serve that purpose.

In order to gain a clearer understanding of the condition for which you want to use a drug, we recommend that you read *Discussion and Cautions,* before you refer to the listing of the various products. Also you should read the chapter entitled "About Side Effects" and Appendix B before actually using any drug.

To facilitate finding the information in this book without obliging the reader to go through a whole chapter devoted to a particular symptom or condition, we have prepared tables headed "If Your Need Is . . ." Ready reference can be made to such a table for a *condensed overview* of what ingredients are best to use for a given condition. These tables are found toward the end of each chapter immediately preceding the section *Names of Products,* which lists the available products and their ingredients. The ingredients in these tables are listed in approximately descending order of preference.

Nonetheless, for a more comprehensive understanding of the subject we suggest you read the whole chapter devoted to a given condition or discomfort.

The listing of products headed *Names of Products* is merely a guide; it gives the name of the product, its manufacturer, and the ingredients it contains—little else. We organized the book in that fashion deliberately: our intention was to give as much useful information as practicable for the layman's use, yet to avoid even an appearance of bias in favor of any product. We strongly believe that the layman can make an intelligent choice when given the basic facts clearly, and impartially.

We further believe that no information can be valid or useful unless the limitations of self-medication are emphasized. The layman is certainly not in the best position to exercise differential judgment—whether a symptom is merely a discomfort or a harbinger of a condition that requires professional treatment. The *caveats* under *Discussion and Cautions* attempt to make him aware that such are the facts of life.

Many disease conditions or even some discomforts will not be found in the table of contents nor in the index. That is also intentional: they are simply not amenable to self-medication because they require either diagnosis or treatment by a physician—or both. This, we believe, is consistent with the practical purpose of the book—to help the reader make an informed and intelligent choice of medicines that he can reasonably safely use by self-medication. To enter into a discourse on other aspects of drugs, or other facets of medicine, would be tangential.

Here is an example of what we mean: although we discuss antacids in some length, to enable you to choose a product for the relief of temporary discomforts, you should not treat your own stomach ulcer, even if you know that antacids are a part of its treatment. A key is in the phrase "a part." Many other aspects, in addition to the use of antacids, must be considered by a physician in the adequate and comprehensive treatment of stomach ulcer. It is not a simple matter of matching ulcer with antacid, nor, on a larger framework, of matching symptom and drug.

THE COMMON COLD

DEFINITION

A cold is a temporary condition of intense discomfort with its characteristic symptoms in the nose, throat, and chest. It is accompanied by a general feeling of ill-being. It is also known as an upper respiratory infection, acute catarrhal rhinitis, coryza, acute nasal catarrh with discharge of mucus from nostrils. All these are more or less synonymous.

CAUSE

Viral infection.

DISCUSSION AND CAUTIONS

A common cold may follow exposure to cold and wet weather, or it may be transmitted by an individual who has a cold. A cold is a viral infection, by and large, or it may be an allergy and show most of the symptoms of a cold. But to people who have a cold it seems that a cold just happens—and they are sure that the first cold of the year comes at almost a given week in the late fall. While some people do get colds during the summer—which may well be allergic happenings—the immense proportion of colds, perhaps 90% of them, occur in a period beginning with November and ending with April.

And a cold does not confer immunity against succeeding

bouts. Often a person who claims he has one cold "lasting all winter" has more likely had a succession of colds with reinfections that perpetuate it.

Colds are characterized by a number of symptoms, though not everyone has all the symptoms. There is usually a low fever; a feeling of chilliness which warmth cannot seem to overcome or a sense of inner heat from which one cannot seem to get relief; a feeling of general malaise better described as feeling "blah"; mild pain in the back or legs, an acute congestion of the nose, usually beginning with dryness and soon developing into a running nose with its characteristic copious, thin or viscid nasal discharge; congestion hence swelling of the nasal mucous membrane; difficulty in breathing due to blocking of the nasal passages; a general feeling of a "stuffed head" to the extent that one's voice does not sound normal; and often laryngitis, i.e., an inflammation of the throat at the voice box.

As if this were not enough discomfort there are often other symptoms suggestive of, or indicative of, congestion in the chest. Therewith, there is cough and, in fact, difficulty in bringing up mucus because it is not yet ready to be expelled.

But the gods are kind. Some people are spared a sore throat. Others begin with a sore throat (pharyngitis) and run through most or all of the symptoms just mentioned. Pharyngitis is an inflammation of the pharynx—the membrane and muscles that lie at the junction of the nasal passage, mouth, and the food pipe or esophagus. Pharyngitis causes pain on swallowing—in fact, even on breathing. This, however, is to be distinguished from its first cousin, laryngitis, which is an inflammation of the voice box, or larynx. Laryngitis produces hoarseness of the voice and difficulty in speaking as well as in swallowing. Since there is dryness and irritation of the mucous membrane, it may also produce a cough. Tonsillitis is an inflammation of the tonsils, with attendant pain on swallowing.

There are many myths regarding the origin and "cure" of colds. Since we know so little about that aspect of colds, they may possibly not be myths—we do not know. One is that a shower or bath in the morning before going outdoors reduces body temperature and produces a cold; another, washing hair and not drying it before going outdoors; third, being exposed to the north wind. In addition, standing in a draft which reduces body temperature is said to produce a cold, and this may not be a myth at all; under these circumstances the body is not merely exposed to surface cold, but is continuously exposed to a cold draft without a chance of recovery of one's normal body temperature. And cold is known as a stressor agent; our natural resistance is embarrassed by exposure to stress.

The question of whether colds turn to pneumonia is still unresolved, though people can certainly get viral pneumonia, but pneumonia is also caused by other organisms. Certainly every cold does not turn into pneumonia. Nonetheless, an infection may extend and may get worse through carelessness and may infect the middle ear, through vigorous nose blowing.

Perhaps a greater number of people suffer colds than any other disease. Colds spare no one, regardless of age, sex, state of health, condition of servitude—high or low estate.

It is therefore not extraordinary to note that there are perhaps more remedies for colds than for any other discomfort or disease. The phrase "what's-good-for-a-cold" has become a form of speech—if laryngitis allows the sufferer to speak.

Remedies are not limited to the conventional drugs. They range from whiskey through hot baths, cold baths, lemon, nutmeg, bed rest, hot honey or heated wheatgerm, vitamins, running to "get-up-a-sweat," to the plethora of drugs.

We are limiting our discussion to drugs, especially those obtainable over-the-counter without a doctor's prescription. But before we discuss those drugs—their similarities as well as their differences—we should make certain comments that apply to all of them:

1. There is no cure for the common cold—remedies merely relieve symptoms to make the cold bearable.
2. If a cold must run its course—according to the folk be-

lief—it is nonetheless reasonable to use some medication in order to ease discomforts during that course.

3. If there is high fever—i.e., more than 101° F in adults or children, especially if it persists for more than 2 days—a physician should be consulted.
4. If a sore throat persists for more than 2 days, a physician should be consulted. This may be a strep throat, which can possibly lead to rheumatic fever, especially in children, or to a kidney inflammation (glomerulonephritis) in adults or children.
5. Do not take antibiotics which a well-meaning friend may offer with the joyous story that it-cured-my-cold-in-no-time. Antibiotics do not kill viruses, to which a cold is due. Antibiotics, while extremely valuable, should be reserved for when needed for serious infections, as taking them casually may cause microorganisms to become accustomed or resistant to them.
6. In case of cold, it is desirable, if possible, to rest in bed, at least for the first day or two. We do not know how bed rest works, except that it increases resistance, but empirically it appears to prevent complications and may possibly reduce the length of time that a cold persists. During a cold, it is wise to take plenty of fluids and citrus juices. Perhaps the best reason for that is that, once again empirically, citrus fruit juices, possibly due to vitamin C content, have been found helpful.
7. Drugs for a cold should be taken as long as the symptoms last—but no longer. In fact, even if symptoms persist or if a cold gets worse, at the end of 10 days a physician should be consulted.
8. It may be necessary to change the medication during a cold for the following reason: if you are taking a product containing a combination of an analgesic with a nasal decongestant and the congestion in the nasal passages clears up, switch to aspirin or some other product not combined with a decongestant if the decongestant keeps you awake or if you have high blood pressure.

A cold has a diversity of symptoms, and its self-treatment by the layman with drugs available over-the-counter without prescription is symptomatic. It follows that a variety of drugs, each one directed to a different group of symptoms, are used to gain some comfort.

For that reason, one or more of the following groups of drugs are used in the attempt to ameliorate the discomforts associated with colds: (1) analgesics, (2) decongestants, (3) antihistamines, and (4) expectorants or cough suppressants.

ANALGESICS

These products do not cure a cold, but they ameliorate some symptoms, such as headache and pain associated with it; and some, as aspirin, salicylamide, or acetaminophen, reduce fever. The oldest and best-known example of this type is aspirin; next are APC tablets, consisting of aspirin, phenacetin and caffeine; then the buffered preparations, which are aspirin buffered with antacids, such as aluminum-magnesium hydroxides. Buffering in this context means the reduction of the acidity of aspirin; aluminum hydroxide, magnesium oxide, hydroxide or carbonate, and even calcium carbonate are used for that purpose.

Within the last several years two new analgesics have appeared on the market and are used broadly. They are (1) acetaminophen (*N*-acetylparaaminophenol; acetylaminophenol; APAP; NAPAP—the last four names are synonyms for acetaminophen) and (2) salicylamide. Whereas salicylamide is a salicylate, like aspirin, acetaminophen belongs to a different group, the paraaminophenols. (While the name *phenol* is a synonym for carbolic acid, do not feel apprehensive about acetaminophen—it is not carbolic acid.) Acetphenetidin, or phenacetin—long an ingredient in APC tablets (aspirin, phenacetin, caffeine)—also belongs to the same group, i.e., it is a member of the paraaminophenols.

There are differences of opinion as to the advantage of

acetaminophen or salicylamide as compared to aspirin. Essentially they have the same pain-relieving or analgesic effect, and a fever-reducing or antipyretic effect. But the antiinflammatory effect of aspirin is pronounced, that of salicylamide is good, while acetaminophen does not have an antiinflammatory effect. The antiinflammatory effect is of especial advantage in the treatment of such conditions as rheumatoid arthritis or other inflammatory conditions. But these are not subjects for treatment by over-the-counter preparations. (See *Arthritis* in the chapter on pain for further discussion.)

Acetphenetidin or phenacetin has been the subject of numerous reports citing its toxic effect on the kidneys. While this is a real danger in its excessive and long-continued use, the sporadic, occasional use, in the moderate doses of phenacetin that are found in those analgesics that contain it, as in APC tablets, carries no significant danger. Nonetheless, those products carry a caution, demanded by the FDA, which reads: "This medication may damage the kidneys when used in large amounts or for too long a period of time. Do not take more than the recommended dosage, nor take regularly for longer than 10 days, without consulting your physician."

On the whole, aspirin or the APC-type tablets are reasonably safe and effective preparations for most people to use to treat the painful discomfort or fever of the common cold. While aspirin does not have the drawback that is associated with APC tablets, which contain phenacetin, aspirin should be used cautiously in people with asthma, because some of them may be sensitive to aspirin. Then there are some, perhaps a small number of people, including children, who may have an unsuspected allergic reaction to aspirin involving a reduction in platelet count, which could expose them to the risk of bleeding difficult to control.

Another point of caution regarding aspirin should be observed by people who are taking oral anticoagulants, which are often prescribed following heart attacks or phlebitis, the latter an inflammation of the lining of the veins where clots form. (Anticoagulants are taken to lessen the coagulability of the blood, in the attempt to prevent heart attacks which result from the formation of blood clots.) People who are taking anticoagulants should not take aspirin *at all.* The reason is that aspirin lessens the coagulability of blood, though mildly. When taken conjointly with oral anticoagulants, aspirin accentuates their anticoagulant effect. Hemorrhage may result. It is difficult enough to assure the safe use of anticoagulants; the problem should not be increased by adding aspirin. To control hemorrhage at a site to which one has no ready access is a risky business. Therefore, people who take anticoagulants but need a mild analgesic or antipyretic can take a product that contains salicylamide or acetaminophen, or even phenacetin, but not aspirin.

Aspirin has another point of caution: it may cause some bleeding in the stomach by damaging the stomach wall. While this is not a general or an invariable problem, it must be considered, especially in people who have stomach ulcer or inflammation of the mucous membrane of the stomach (gastritis), or those whose alcoholic consumption in the past has perhaps given them a chronic alcoholic gastritis. Another caution: people often take aspirin, among other measures, to overcome the headache or other discomforts of an alcoholic hangover. Don't.

In fact, chronic aspirin takers at times have baffling bleeding conditions which may be due to taking huge or even just large or overfrequent doses of aspirin. This does not mean that aspirin should not be taken, when needed, for conditions that are susceptible to relief by aspirin.

However, it does mean that if you have or have had a stomach ulcer, or gastritis, or frequent stomach upsets, you will do better with salicylamide or acetaminophen, or perhaps phenacetin, particularly in nursing a hangover.

However, should you find that aspirin is the drug that gives you relief, rather than salicylamide or acetaminophen, you should keep the following points in mind:

1. Never take aspirin after—or before—alcohol.
2. Take it with food, or with a glassful of milk, or with a tablespoonful of an aluminum-magnesium liquid antacid.

(Buffered aspirin tablets do not contain enough of the antacid to serve the same purpose.)

3. Or take aspirin in the form of an effervescent drink. This is made by dropping effervescent tablets into water and drinking the liquid after most of the effervescence has subsided. These products contain aspirin with other ingredients, notably sodium bicarbonate and citric acid. As a result, the aspirin is converted into a sodium salt of aspirin, which is not acidic, as in the case with aspirin. It is not yet clear whether the acid reaction of aspirin or another factor is responsible in producing the bleeding in many gastritic stomachs. Incidentally, in effervescent solution aspirin is more rapidly absorbed and probably works faster, but commensurately its effect is more rapidly dissipated, as compared with an aspirin tablet. (If you must restrict your intake of sodium, due to high blood pressure or for other reasons, be aware that the effervescent products do contain a small amount of sodium, from the sodium bicarbonate.)

The following table outlines the similarities and differences among aspirin, salicylamide, acetaminophen and phenacetin:

Effects	*Aspirin*	*Salicylamide*	*Acetaminophen*	*Phenacetin*
Onset of pain relief	Rapid	Rapid	Less rapid	Less rapid
Duration	Average	Average	Longer	Longer
Reduce fever?	Yes	Yes	Yes	No
Reduce inflammation?	Yes	Yes	No	No
Suitable to take in aspirin sensitivity?	No	Yes	Yes	Yes
Cause possible stomach bleeding?	Yes	No	No	No
Suitable to take when on anticoagulants?	No	Yes	Yes	Yes

Note: Such factors as rapidity and duration of pain relief are reasonable approximations and cannot be expressed as absolute factors.

DECONGESTANTS

Since the common cold has a variety of symptoms, and the form of treatment is largely symptomatic, it follows that preparations having effects additional to that of analgesics are used. Among them are decongestants and antihistamines, which are often used orally, usually in combination with aspirin or in the APC type preparations. Decongestants are also available in the form of nose drops or sprays.

The decongestants found in over-the-counter preparations include salts of phenylephrine, phenylpropanolamine, ephedrine, possibly certain other ephedrine derivatives as desoxyephedrine, also naphazoline, and methoxyphenamine. The same ingredients are used in oral decongestant tablets as well as in sprays, drops, or jellies for application into the nostrils. There is virtually no difference in effect among hydrochlorides, sulfates, tartrates, etc., of the above decongestants; these salts merely make the decongestants water-soluble.

During colds, the nostrils are largely affected in one of two ways: (a) they run, which is due to an inflammation of the mucous membrane inside the nostrils, or (b) they are congested, which is due to the swelling or congestion of the inflamed membrane of the nostrils, which prevents breathing through the nose.

Our discussion here is centered on stuffy or running nose in colds. However, it must be borne in mind that unless associated with a cold, there are numerous reasons for nostrils being stuffy or even running. For example, is it only one nostril that feels clogged up? If this is customary it may be due to an anatomical obstruction or even a foreign body. If both sides are affected and it is chronic and recurrent, it may be due to allergy, sinusitis, nervous nose running (vasomotor rhinitis), or simply infection.

The term *rhinitis* refers to an inflammation of the mucous membrane of the nostrils. The symptoms may be running nose or stuffy nose. The term *rhinorrhea* means running nose. The term *nasal congestion* commonly encompasses both, though strictly it means stuffy nose.

Among symptoms of the common cold are congested or running nose in which there is a discharge of thin or viscid mucus. Decongestants make breathing easier if the difficulty of breathing is due to stuffy nose. They do so by shrinking the engorged, swollen mucous membrane of the nose, allowing air to pass through the nose, and thus they facilitate breathing more easily. The shrinking process also lessens somewhat, at least transiently, the discharge of the thin mucus, but it does not get rid of mucus. Decongestants are no cure, merely temporary relief of nasal congestion or sinuslike symptoms, which obviously is welcome. But decongestants are not a cure for an inflammation of the sinuses either, though they are properly prescribed in sinusitis or inflammation of the sinuses.

It is better not to take decongestants late in the evening as in some people they may produce wakefulness. When taken orally—either alone or combined with an APC-like tablet—they are more effective, as they are distributed by the circulation of the blood, and their effect may last longer.

Decongestants work by reducing congestion in nostrils, eustachian tube in the ear, sinuses and bronchi.

Decongestants may also be used in the form of a solution (drops or preferably sprays) or a jelly for application into the nostrils. These have certain advantages and disadvantages. One advantage is that application into the nostrils may give a more rapid effect, though it does not last as long as when the decongestant is taken orally. A disadvantage is that if the nasal mucus is viscid or thick, the drops will not touch the swollen membrane, as the mucus forms an effective barrier. The taking of oral decongestants while using decongestant nose sprays may have additive effects, possibly resulting in a larger dose than commonly advisable, but it will usually do no harm to use the drops judiciously at the time one needs most relief, while taking the oral decongestants.

As to the difference among decongestants in spray, drop or jelly form, the advantage seems to lie in sprays and then drops. The reason is that sprays or drops, being aqueous, carry a greater likelihood of bringing the medication in contact with mucous membrane. A jelly, though it is water-miscible, may merely cover the debris in the nose, or may be washed out by the discharging nostrils, before it has a chance to work.

Nose drops that have an oil base are still available. We do not recommend their use at all. There are two reasons: one is a matter of safety in that the possible inhalation of particles of oil droplets may set up an irritation in the lungs and in extreme cases, especially when the head is tilted back while the drops are put in, may lead to fat pneumonia or lipid pneumonia. The second is a matter of efficacy: a water-based solution makes better contact with the mucous membrane which is discharging mucus.

ANTIHISTAMINES

Some of the symptoms of allergy, such as running nose, resemble those of the common cold. Therefore it was believed that the common cold, though an infection, may have an allergic component.

Hence, preparations for the common cold arose which contained in addition to aspirin or the APC formula, with or without a decongestant, a small amount of an antihistamine. The antihistamines are added to aspirin, or more commonly to APC combinations or to other combinations with decongestants.

Thus we have products that contain analgesics-decongestants-antihistamines. Since they minister to the variety of symptoms of the common cold, they are a convenient form to take in the attempt to moderate its symptoms. It appears that the antihistamines do perform a desirable function, although well-controlled universally satisfactory tests comparing them to those combinations without antihistamines have not been available; in fact, there is considerable doubt if they can actually be done meaningfully.

The amount of antihistamines in the tablets used for the

treatment of the common cold is smaller than the doses of the same antihistamines used in the treatment of allergy *per se.* For example, one popular product contains 2 mg. chlorpheniramine per tablet. That amount is allowed for sale over-the-counter. Tablets of chlorpheniramine alone, containing 4 mg. chlorpheniramine, are available only on prescription. Paradoxically, a dose of two tablets used for the treatment of the common cold, each 2 mg. chlorpheniramine, will contain 4 mg. chlorpheniramine, but is safe to take, without prescription, if taken according to directions.

Other antihistamines in products for the treatment of common cold are phenindamine, phenyltoloxamine, or pyrilamine.

The antihistamines are used in the form of salts, such as maleate, hydrochloride, tartrate, citrate, etc. There is virtually no difference in effect among these salts; they merely make the antihistamines water-soluble.

While there are differences in degree of effects or side effects among the variety of antihistamines, it is not generally possible to predict which one is preferable for the common cold. It is largely a matter of individual reaction. However, some antihistamines produce a greater degree of sleepiness as a side effect, particularly methapyrilene and pyrilamine. (For that reason they are used principally in over-the-counter sleeping remedies.) Since antihistamines tend to make most users somewhat drowsy, or relaxed, they should not be taken, alone or in combination, when alertness is required, as when driving a car.

But decongestants, as a side effect, produce the opposite, i.e., varying degrees of wakefulness, especially if taken at or near bedtime. Thus the antihistamines serve a double purpose: (a) they confer whatever comfort they do in ameliorating the symptoms of the common cold, and (b) they minimize, or may negate by their drowsiness-producing effect, the stimulation or wakefulness provided by the decongestants. And the reverse is also true: the stimulating effect of the decongestants reduces the sleep-producing effect of the antihistamines.

For these reasons, assuming that the symptoms of the common cold are multiple at a given time in a given individual, it is preferable to take a combination product, containing an analgesic-decongestant-antihistamine combination.

However, should there not be a stuffy or running nose in a common cold at a given time, no decongestant is necessary.

What about vitamin C, or ascorbic acid, increasingly used in tablets containing a combination of ingredients for the common cold? Ascorbic acid is not an analgesic, nor decongestant nor antihistaminic. But many people find, or at least believe, that ascorbic acid is comforting to them when taken in the presence of symptoms. And there is a rationale for this belief: vitamin C is useful in stress, as during stress there is a depletion of vitamin C.

Predictably, there are a number of tablets for the treatment of cold symptoms that contain ascorbic acid. But if it is advisable to take ascorbic acid, it should be taken in doses of about 1,000 mg. (1 gm.) a day. The cold tablets do not contain enough. It is simpler to take 250 mg. tablets of ascorbic acid 3 to 4 times a day, together or apart from the cold tablets.

There are often reasons for taking a preparation—in this case ascorbic acid as a supplement to cold tablets—despite the fact that there is no incontrovertible evidence for its usefulness. But in conditions such as a common cold when there are no incontrovertible remedies (and what remedies are incontrovertible?) it is logical indeed to take a product that, while there is no hard evidence to support it, (a) is safe, and (b) there is sufficient *empirical* evidence to suggest the wisdom of using it.

EXPECTORANTS AND COUGH SUPPRESSANTS

A cough may be one of the symptoms of the common cold. Or a cough may develop during any stage of a cold.

Coughs frequently serve a useful purpose. When a foreign body enters the respiratory tract the cough reflex triggers a cough in the attempt to expel it, to maintain the unencumbered freedom of the passage of air and secretions. A cough may also be a significant diagnostic sign pointing to another or a more serious condition, such as heart disease, an obstruction as a new growth in or near the respiratory tract, a postnasal drip or disease of the lungs. The coughs of tuberculosis or typhoid fever, for example, are well known.

We can recognize a cough, which is a forceful expulsion of air, when we hear one. Since they come in various sizes and types, they have modifying names. Here is a condensed glossary defining some of the terms relating to coughs:

productive cough	one that produces phlegm or mucus which comes up with coughing.
nonproductive cough	a dry cough, producing no mucus.
reflex cough	a cough that is a result of a disturbance or irritation, which may not at all be associated with the respiratory tract; it may originate in the vocal cords, the ear, or even the stomach.
bronchitis	an inflammation of the bronchial tubes, usually associated with a cough.
sputum	this is *not* saliva, but the material that is coughed up, commonly called phlegm or mucus.
croup	a combination of symptoms in the respiratory tract during which there is difficulty in breathing, much mucus, and a spasm of the voice box or larynx; it may or may not be associated with a cough, but the objective is to produce a cough to expel the accumulation. So-called croupy cough is usually not croup, but a cough with much phlegm.
expectorant	a medicinal agent that aids in the expulsion of phlegm and other mucus from the respiratory tract.

Another type of cough is an attention-getting cough. People have many ways of calling attention to themselves: they can scream and spit; do bizarre tricks; overcompensate for a real or fancied deficiency; pollute the atmosphere by producing rock music; use four-letter words where it will be shocking; wet their pants, in the case of children. They may cough. The attention-getting cough is a small, dry cough, which begins a sentence or even punctuates it. Drugs are not for that cough. What such people need is attention. All of us compete for the attention of others and the more aggressive or self-sufficient are more likely to get it. The others use different means to gain attention—including a cough. In many respects, such a cough may be as involuntary as a tic. This is called a nervous cough.

While we are primarily concerned with coughs that are associated with the common cold or are sequels to them, we should point out briefly that the general treatment of cough is not merely an ameliorative step to make the person coughing more comfortable. A cough can literally be a lifesaver when it clears the airway. An impeded airway can be life-threatening. A cough clears the airway as it may drain the air passages in the bronchial branches. A cough can be lifesaving when there is a great deal of bronchial debris or sputum to dispose of. It is as important to cough up such debris as it is to cough up a swallowed coin.

Under certain conditions, as after anesthesia or as an effect of such drugs as opium or barbiturates, the cough reflex may be depressed and a person can drown in his own bronchial secretions. There are other conditions in which it may be difficult to cough, as when the muscles that help the explosive cough phenomenon are inhibited. Such conditions occur after a stroke, in polio, or in a condition in which muscle reaction is weak, as in myasthenia gravis, in which there is a neuromuscular depression taking strength and function from muscles.

What is expelled? Predominantly sputum or mucus, which is an abundant secretion that forms in mucous membrane as a response to irritation or inflammation. Thick mucus is more dangerous, as it may act as a solid plug which stops air intake. One of the objectives in cough preparations is to help make the thick mucus thinner to help expel it—to make the cough *productive.*

(A part of the mechanism of cough production can be likened to an internal combustion engine of a car, which takes in air, compresses it by valves, then forces it out; the air rushing out supplies the motive power. Similarly in a cough, air is sucked into the lungs, it is compressed when the top of the windpipe, the glottis, momentarily closes, then the compressed air is released with an explosive force.)

In most instances of the common cold there is irritation of the bronchi or irritation and tickling of the pharynx, leading to cough. In treating a cough due to the common cold, there are two objectives: (a) to give comfort by expelling sputum or mucus through a productive cough, and (b) to depress the cough reflex. In many instances sedatives are added to a cough preparation to attain the second objective, i.e., to reduce the irritability of the mucous membrane and to reduce the cough reflex in the brain, thus mitigating the violent paroxysms of coughs.

A cough preparation does not prevent coughs if taken in advance, even those resulting from the common cold. It does not even cure such a cold—it merely liquefies tenacious phlegm aiding its expulsion, or it soothes tickling of the throat which produces a cough. When these functions are completed the cough ceases. Coughs lasting longer than a week or 10 days or associated with fever, shortness of breath or bloody sputum should not be self-medicated but a physician should be consulted.

Among expectorants for making a cough productive are ammonium chloride, terpin hydrate, glyceryl guaiacolate, potassium iodide, syrup of ipecac, syrup of squill, sodium citrate, and volatile oils such as that of eucalyptus or the solid part of oil of peppermint, which is menthol. Among the above, glyceryl guaiacolate has many advantages in that it is an effective expectorant and does not upset the stomach. Terpin hydrate is probably as effective, though it may more likely cause some stomach upset. Ammonium chloride is also an excellent expectorant. Potassium iodide thins mucus but it should not be used by people who have thyroid disease. Expectorants are not strictly cough suppressants but stimulate the production of a thinner mucus to enable it to be brought up, expectorated.

True cough suppressants actually have a sedative effect. They reduce the sensitivity of the cough reflex, making it somewhat less responsive, thereby reducing the cough. In larger doses they also depress respiration or more severely depress the cough reflex, restraining the expulsion of sputum or mucus. Codeine, in addition to offering pain relief, is the most effective cough suppressant. In the small amounts used for over-the-counter sale, without a prescription—i.e., 65 mg. (1 grain) per 1 oz. of the phosphate or sulfate when used in teaspoonful (5 cc) doses—there is little danger of habit formation. But it may be constipating—a small price to pay for cough relief.

Noscapine is not a narcotic and does not depress respiration; it works by a different mechanism, i.e., as an antispasmodic, by reducing spasm. It is not constipating, nor pain-relieving, but is an effective cough suppressant. Dextromethorphan hydrobromide is not a narcotic, is also similar to codeine in its effect but is not constipating, and is probably the most available of cough suppressants.

In treating coughs as a symptom of a common cold, it is good judgment to try first a product containing dextromethorphan, before taking a codeine preparation, because it is easier to get preparations with effective doses of dextromethorphan than with codeine. If the dextromethorphan preparation does not mitigate the cough, a codeine preparation can be used.

In attempting to reduce or suppress the cough associated with the common cold, it is highly advisable to take a preparation or mixture containing both an expectorant and a cough suppressant. The reason is based on the premise that the objective is *both* to cause an expulsion of sputum or mucus (expectorant) as well as to reduce the severity of the cough paroxysm (cough suppressant). For dry cough use a cough suppressant. For productive coughs use an expectorant with or without a suppressant.

Cough preparations often contain, in addition to expectorants and cough suppressants, decongestants such as salts of phenylpropanolamine, phenylephrine, or ephedrine. They are often a welcome addition, since they dilate the bronchial capillaries, thus reducing bronchoconstriction, which is one phase of the cough reflex. They also have a decongestive effect, reducing a postnasal drip which can add to the problem of triggering a cough reflex. Many cough preparations also contain an antihistamine. The roles of decongestants and antihistamines in the symptomatic treatment of colds has been described earlier in this chapter.

Lozenges or Troches: These are tablets that are intended to be held in the mouth to relieve throat irritation and to reduce the stimulus that tickling contributes to coughs and colds. They usually contain an antiseptic, like cetylpyridinium chloride or hexylresorcinol. They are not an adequate treatment of the symptoms of colds or coughs, but they have an advantage in that they tend to keep the throat moist, reducing the irritation arising from dryness. An exception to the above are lozenges which do contain dextromethorphan, a cough suppressant, and benzyl alcohol, which acts as a mild local anesthetic somewhat reducing the tickling sensation.

Many myths have arisen regarding coughs. It may be interesting to consider them.

Myth 1: The following was written by Sir William Osler in 1892, one of the giants of medicine: "The hot foot-bath, or the warm bath, a drink of hot lemonade, and a mustard plaster on the chest will often give relief. . . . Relief is obtained from the unpleasant sense of rawness by keeping the air of the room saturated with moisture. . . . For the cough, when dry and irritating, opium should be freely used." Today, Osler would be accused of starting a drug culture by his recommendation of using opium freely—the authorities would want to know who his pusher is. But keeping the air moist is a good idea—provided that it is not kept moist with opium.

Myth 2: Honey alone or honey and milk are said to be specific remedies for coughs. Milk may well be helpful; it is a demulcent for irritated throats. What about honey? Honey may be superb for the attention-getting cough, especially if given to the sufferer by his own honey if he has one. He can use some attention. In fact, milk, soda, soup, hot or even cold water should serve equally well—if attention is paid to the cougher. But it must be given especially kindly, with soothing words, and not with recriminations such as "anybody-knows-enough-not-to-go-out-without-rubbers." Such a reminder can make both the cough and the nerves raw. Almost anything given tenderly to the attention-getting cougher may unpredictably cure him.

There are many myths connected with the common cold. Some actually work! The myths that worked every time are:

Myth 1: Wear a garlic clove around the neck. This myth pays dividends as the people wearing garlic are less prone to infection—because no one will come near them to spray them with cold germs.

Myth 2: Put on a mustard plaster because it burns hell out of cold germs. This is another useful myth—because you have to go to bed after being mustard-plastered. The rest in bed is great for colds.

Myth 3: Scotch or bourbon whiskey straight is both antiseptic and stimulates circulation which breaks up a cold. This is not a myth but a rationalization for an alcoholic. Perhaps that is the reason alcoholics sit on drafty stools at bars to get a cold, in order to be able to take the cure. In fact, they have even named a beer after it—draft beer. But there may be something to it: whiskey dilates blood vessels, and dilating those of the nose increases the amount of mucus. Yet, the depressing effect of whiskey, any alcohol, is what a person with a cold can do without.

INGREDIENTS

The following ingredients are all analgesics: aspirin, salicylamide, acetaminophen, and phenacetin. (For details see under *Discussion and Cautions* on pages 23–27.)

The following ingredients are all decongestants:

Phenylpropanolamine Hydrochloride (Propadrine)
Phenylephrine Hydrochloride (Neo-Synephrine)
Methoxyphenamine Hydrochloride (Orthoxine)
Ephedrine Hydrochloride or Sulfate
Naphazoline Hydrochloride (Privine)
Xylometazoline Hydrochloride (Otrivin)

They are common ingredients in cold tablets or cough mixtures, reducing the engorged mucous membrane of the nostrils to allow passage of air. Their side effects are wakefulness, increase in blood pressure, and acceleration of the heartbeat (tachycardia). But there is little likelihood of these side effects, in the small amounts they are used, both per tablet or per spray if used as a nasal spray. However, they should not be used in doses greater than recommended on the labels. Another use to which these ingredients are put is to relieve the difficulties of breathing in bronchial asthma, as they relax bronchial muscles (while they constrict capillaries in the mucous membrane of the nostrils).

The following ingredients are all antihistamines:

Thonzylamine Hydrochloride (Anahist)
Phenyltoloxamine Citrate (Bristamin)
Phenindamine Tartrate (Thephorin)
Chlorpheniramine Maleate (Chlor-Trimeton)
Pyrilamine Maleate (Neo-Antergan)
Thenyldiamine Hydrochloride (Thenfadil)
Methapyrilene Fumarate (Histadyl)
Doxylamine Succinate (Decapryn)

They are common ingredients in "cold tablets" or cough mixtures. The reason for their inclusion rests on the idea of ministering to the allergic component of the cold or cough, to confer comfort from symptoms. A common side effect is drowsiness, and it is not possible to tell which one produces less drowsiness or, in fact, which is a more effective and preferable one. One of the reasons is that different individuals respond differently to each of them. In some, in the doses found in over-the-counter products (for example, chlorpheniramine), sleep is induced, whereas in others it does not even make a person drowsy. The ones most commonly used in over-the-counter products available without a prescription are chlorpheniramine and methapyrilene. It can be assumed that for that reason—their broad use—they have fewest side effects, but there is no certainty of that. Another useful purpose the antihistamines serve is in relaxing the individual, due to their drowsiness-producing effect.

The amount of each ingredient is given if it appears on the label. Usually, all are comparable, because due to FDA policy there is a limit of the quantities that a product may contain and be suitable for over-the-counter sale without a prescription.

The following ingredients are for coughs: dextromethorphan hydrobromide and glyceryl guaiacolate.

Modern cough mixtures usually contain dextromethorphan hydrobromide as a cough suppressant—a good choice. Antihistamines, as well as decongestants, are present for the same reason as in decongestive cold tablets.

Glyceryl guaiacolate, a frequently used ingredient in cough mixtures, is an expectorant, increasing the quantity of fluid in the respiratory tract, thus reducing viscosity of sputum or mucus so as to expel it easier. Potassium guaiacol sulfonate is used for the same purpose but with lesser effect.

Many cough mixtures contain small amounts of chloroform, probably intended for its soothing effect. It is, however, not of much use because most of the little quantity present evaporates quickly after the bottle is opened. The presence of alcohol is not for the amelioration of the cough; it is there as a solvent for some of the other ingredients. (The reason that the quantities of chloroform and alcohol are invariably given on the label is because of a federal law that requires a statement of proportion of certain substances, among which are chloroform and alcohol. It is not because they are important cough-relieving ingredients.)

Sodium citrate is a mild expectorant, but its effect is dubious for that purpose. Ammonium chloride, found in some cough preparations, is a good expectorant.

However, some cough preparations, long on the market, contain such ingredients as white pine, blood root, wild cherry, squill, ipecac, oil of eucalyptus, glycerophosphates, creosote. None of these is favored now, and in fact the more modern preparations containing dextromethorphan and glyceryl guaiacolate are more functional. Ipecac is intended to bring up sputum; it is also an emetic. Creosote is a fine antiseptic, but its usefulness in a cough mixture is now questionable. White pine and wild cherry, favorites of a generation ago, will do no harm but are not expected to do good.

INHALERS

Inhalers as well as drops intended for nasal congestion are available. The inhalers are small rigid tubes which are inhaled while held under the nose; the vapor they contain is drawn up into the nose to reduce the swollen, congested membrane. The active ingredient is usually propylhexedrine. This is a successor to the Benzedrine Inhalers which were withdrawn from over-the-counter sale; propylhexedrine does not have the strong effect of Benzedrine or amphetamine. These inhalers also contain menthol, which lends a cooling sensation with the aim of increasing comfort. Menthol is not a decongestant.

Other preparations called nasal sprays are packed in plastic squeeze bottles which deliver a spurt of spray into the nose when held under the nose and squeezed. They contain one or more of the following preparations: phenylephrine hydrochloride, naphazoline hydrochloride, phenylpropanolamine hydrochloride, which are nasal decongestants. They are usually effective in shrinking the engorged nasal mucous membrane and allowing one to breathe through the nostril.

Some of the nasal sprays also contain pyrilamine maleate, methapyrilene hydrochloride, or chlorpheniramine gluconate. These substances are antihistamines included with the aim of making breathing comfortable if the nasal congestion is due to allergy or if there is an allergic component to the common cold. The whole objective of these nasal decongestants, in whatever form, is to reduce nasal congestion and make breathing easier.

That they do. The relief may, however, be short-lived and may last from 15 minutes to an hour or somewhat more.

However, naphazoline hydrochloride has a stronger central nervous system effect, and should not be used in children because of its depressing effect. Phenylpropanolamine hydrochloride has much less of this effect.

Most of the decongestants should not be used before bedtime, as they may possibly cause sleeplessness in some people.

While they offer comfort, in nasal congestion due to hay fever, rhinitis and sinusitis, they have an intrinsic drawback if used too frequently: they may cause chronic rhinitis, often called rebound congestion. Rhinitis is exactly what one sets out to relieve.

Other types of preparations for the relief of nasal congestion are nose drops. They do indeed shrink the swollen mucous membrane. But one is in a better position with a spray, as there is a greater likelihood of using more of the nose drops than spray, thus more often producing rebound congestion.

MEDICATED ROOM VAPORIZER

Another form of preparation used in the attempt to mitigate the symptoms of colds is the medicated room vaporizer. This is *not* taken as a medicine. These preparations are used for spraying the air of rooms, presumably to make the person with a cold more comfortable in the room. These vaporizing sprays are called by several modifying names as *medicated room vaporizers, medicated aerosols,* etc. Specifically, these products are aerosols containing certain ingredients which when breathed are intended to have a relieving effect on the cold sufferer.

Inhalation is one of the most effective ways of delivering a medication due to quick and more direct absorption of medication by the bloodstream. But these room vaporizers are intended to spread only a trace of medication in the room itself; they are not for close inhalation by an individual.

The ingredients they contain are much the same as those that are also used in cough mixtures and throat troches—namely menthol, camphor, eucalyptol, and oils such as peppermint, lavender and methyl salicylate. The last three are merely odorants and do not have a medicinal value as used in the aerosols. However, menthol, camphor and eucalyptol, inhaled in minute quantities, do have a cooling, hence comforting effect. They may reduce discomfort of nasal congestion, but they do not have any effect on bronchial congestion.

All of these aerosols also contain triethylene or dipropylene glycols. The glycols resemble glycerine, and they absorb moisture. The reason they are used is because they are toxic to microorganisms, and they keep the air moist, provided they are used in conjunction with a room vaporizer that spreads moisture—water vapor—into the air. Moisture itself is helpful in reducing discomforts when the throat is dry as it so often is when one has a cold.

While the room aerosols, spraying cooling menthol, etc., into the air, are conceivably comforting, they are not anywhere near as effective as cough and cold preparations can be. They are not a substitute for an adequate over-the-counter preparation in relieving the symptoms. The reason lies in the fact that the nature of the medications differs, the amounts of medication are minute, and dilution with air in the spray is prodigal.

These products should not be sprayed close to the nose—they can be dangerous when used that way, due to the propellants they contain, which gives the medicating ingredients the motive power to escape the can in which they are compressed.

PRODUCTS

Except as expressly stated and recommended by us, the list of products given is merely a guide. The ingredients themselves are evaluated in the text. Using that as a guide, you will be able to compare and evaluate what product best serves your purpose. And many products are so similar as to suggest that the reputation of the manufacturer or the price is the really significant factor in the choice to be made.

When the amount of ingredients is listed below the name of the product (if they are given on the label), it refers to the stated amount in one teaspoonful (5cc) in the case of liquids or per tablet in the case of tablets.

Some manufacturers list the amount of ingredients in the old avoirdupois system (grains), but most of them use the much simpler metric system (milligrams, grams). To enable you to compare and to convert, if necessary, here are a few commonly used amounts and conversions:

1 grain (abbreviated *gr.*)	=	64.8 milligrams (abbreviated *mg.*)
1 mg.	=	1/64 grain
1 gram (abbreviated *gm.*)	=	1,000 mg.

Usually the amounts stated are rounded off on the label, justifiably so, to reduce confusion. The conversions below are in terms of rounded-off figures:

15 gr.	=	1,000 mg.	
5 gr.	=	325 mg.	(or 300 mg.)
3½ gr.	=	225 mg.	
3 gr.	=	200 mg.	
2½ gr.	=	150 mg.	
2 gr.	=	130 mg.	
1½ gr.	=	100 mg.	
1 gr.	=	65 mg.	
½ gr.	=	30 mg.	
¼ gr.	=	15 mg.	
⅛ gr.	=	8 mg.	
1/12 gr.	=	5 mg.	

If Your Need Is for a Product Against the Symptoms of the Common Cold:

Look for Products Containing the Following Ingredients:

- Analgesics, as
  - aspirin
  - APC tablets
  - salicylamide
  - acetaminophen
  - phenacetin
- Decongestants, as

phenylephrine
phenylpropanolamine
ephedrine
naphazoline
methoxyphenamine
(the above 5 for oral or nasal use)
propylhexedrine (for inhalation only)

Antihistamines, as
chlorpheniramine
methapyrilene
pyrilamine
phenyltoloxamine
doxylamine
(all are for oral or nasal use)

Expectorants, as
glyceryl guaiacolate
ammonium chloride
terpin hydrate
Avoid syrup of ipecac—a small amount helps expectorant action but in larger amounts it is an emetic.

Cough Suppressants, as
dextromethorphan
codeine
noscapine

Antiseptics in Throat Lozenges, as
cetylpyridinium
benzocaine
hexachlorophene

Avoid the Following Ingredients:
Antibiotics (because colds are viral infections and antibiotics are for bacterial infections)

NAMES OF PRODUCTS

ANALGESICS

Alka-Seltzer Tablets (Miles)—Contains aspirin, monocalcium phosphate, sodium bicarbonate, citric acid; in solution it becomes sodium aspirin, calcium sodium phosphate, sodium bicarbonate, and sodium citrate.

Anacin Tablets (Whitehall)—Contains aspirin and caffeine.

Aspergum (Pharmaco) —Contains aspirin 3½ grains.

Aspirin Tablets (Various Manufacturers) —Contains aspirin 5 grains.

Bayer Aspirin Tablets (Sterling Drug) —Contains aspirin 5 grains.

Bayer Timed-Release Aspirin (Bayer) —Contains aspirin 10 grains.

B.C. Headache Powder (Block Drug) —Contains aspirin, salicylamide, and caffeine.

B.C. Tablets (Block Drug) —Contains aspirin, salicylamide, and caffeine.

Bromo Seltzer (Warner-Lambert) —Each capful contains acetaminophen 3 gr., phenacetin 2 gr., potassium bromide 2½ gr., caffeine, sodium bicarbonate, and citric acid.

Bufferin Tablets (Bristol-Myers) —Contains aspirin 5 gr. with aluminum-magnesium buffers.

Cope Tablets (Glenbrook) —Contains aspirin, methapyrilene fumarate, caffeine, and aluminum-magnesium buffers. (Methapyrilene fumarate is an antihistamine, the side effect of which is drowsiness, hence relaxation.)

Coricidin Tablets (Schering) —Contains chlorpheniramine maleate 2 mg., aspirin 390 mg., and caffeine 30 mg. (Chlorpheniramine is an antihistamine.)

Empirin Compound Tablets (Burroughs Wellcome) —Contains phenacetin 2½ gr., aspirin 3½ gr., and caffeine ½ gr.

Excedrin Tablets (Bristol-Myers) —Contains acetaminophen 1½ gr., salicylamide 2 gr., aspirin 3 gr., and caffeine 1 gr.

Excedrin *PM* Tablets (Bristol-Myers) —Contains APAP 2½ gr., salicylamide, aspirin, methapyrilene fumarate. (Methapyrilene fumarate is an antihistamine, the side effect of which is drowsiness, hence relaxation.)

Fizrin Instant Alkalizer Seltzer (Glenbrook) —Contains aspirin 5 gr., sodium bicarbonate, sodium carbonate, citric acid; in solution it becomes sodium aspirin, sodium bicarbonate, and sodium citrate.

Measurin Timed-Release Aspirin Tablets (Glenbrook) —Contains 10 gr. aspirin.

Nebs Tablets (Eaton) —Contains acetaminophen 325 mg. (5 gr.).

Thephorin-AC Tablets (Roche) —Contains phenindamine tartrate (Thephorin) 10 mg., aspirin 160 mg., phenacetin 160 mg., and caffeine 15 mg. (Phenindamine is an antihistamine.)

Tylenol Tablets (McNeil) —Contains acetaminophen 325 mg. (5 gr.).

Valadol Tablets (Squibb) —Contains acetaminophen 325 mg. (5 gr.).

Vanquish Caplets (Glenbrook)—Contains aspirin 227 mg., acetaminophen 194 mg., caffeine 33 mg., with aluminum-magnesium buffer.

ANALGESIC-DECONGESTANT COMBINATIONS

(Usually with an Antihistamine)

Alka-Seltzer Plus Cold Tablets (Miles)—Contains aspirin, monocalcium phosphate, sodium bicarbonate, phenylephrine, chlorpheniramine, citric acid with vitamin C; in solution it becomes sodium aspirin, calcium sodium phosphate, sodium bicarbonate, sodium citrate, phenylephrine, chlorpheniramine, and vitamin C.

Anahist with Aspirin Tablets (Warner-Lambert)—Contains thonzylamine hydrochloride 6.25 mg., phenyltoloxamine citrate 6.25 mg., phenylpropanolamine hydrochloride 12.5 mg., aspirin 227 mg., phenacetin 97.2 mg., and caffeine.

Bromo Quinine with Laxative (Bristol-Myers)—Contains quinine hydrobromide 25 mg., acetaminophen 100 mg., salicylamide 200 mg., phenylephrine hydrochloride 5 mg., caffeine 15 mg., and yellow phenolphthalein 10 mg. (a laxative).

Cheracol Capsules (Upjohn)—Contains chlorpheniramine maleate 2 mg., orthoxine (methoxyphenamine) hydrochloride 25 mg., aspirin 324 mg., and caffeine anhydrous 32.4 mg.

Contac Capsules (Menley & James)—Contains belladonna alkaloids 0.2 mg., phenylpropanolamine hydrochloride 50 mg., and chlorpheniramine maleate 4 mg.—in timed-disintegration form.

Coricidin D Decongestant Tablets (Schering)—Contains chlorpheniramine maleate 2 mg., phenylephrine 10 mg., aspirin 390 mg., and caffeine 30 mg.

Coryban-D Capsules (Roerig)—Contains salicylamide 230 mg., phenacetin 160 mg., caffeine 30 mg., ascorbic acid 25 mg., chlorpheniramine maleate 2 mg., and phenylpropanolamine hydrochloride 25 mg.

Dristan Decongestant Tablets (Whitehall)—Contains phenylephrine hydrochloride 5 mg., phenindamine tartrate 10 mg., aspirin, caffeine, and aluminum-magesium buffer. (Phenindamine is an antihistamine.)

Dristan 12-Hour Decongestant Capsules (Whitehall)—Contains phenylephrine hydrochloride 20 mg. and chlorpheniramine maleate 4 mg.

Fiogesic Tablets (Sandoz)—Contains aspirin derivative, 382 mg., equivalent to 300 mg. aspirin; phenylpropanolamine hydrochloride, 25 mg.; pheniramine maleate, 12.5 mg.; and pyrilamine maleate, 12.5 mg.

4-Way Cold Tablets (Bristol-Myers)—Contains phenylephrine hydrochloride 5 mg., aspirin, magnesium hydroxide, and yellow phenolphthalein (a laxative).

Neo-Synephrine Compound Cold Tablets (Winthrop)—Contains Neo-Synephrine hydrochloride (phenylephrine hydrochloride) 5 mg., Thenfadil (thenyldiamine) hydrochloride 7.5 mg., acetaminophen 150 mg., and caffeine 15 mg.

NyQuil Liquid (Vick)—One fluid ounce contains acetaminophen 600 mg., ephedrine sulfate, doxylamine succinate, dextromethorphan hydrobromide, and alcohol 25%.

Ornex Decongestant & Analgesic Capsules (Smith Kline & French)—Contains acetaminophen 175 mg., salicylamide 150 mg., caffeine 15 mg., and phenylephrine hydrochloride 18 mg.

Sinarest Tablets (Pharmacraft)—Contains acetaminophen 300 mg., caffeine 30 mg., chlorpheniramine maleate 1 mg., and phenylephrine hydrochloride 5 mg.

Sine-Aid Tablets (Johnson & Johnson)—Contains aspirin, chlorpheniramine maleate, and phenylpropanolamine hydrochloride.

Sine-Off Tablets (Menley & James)—Contains aspirin 325 mg., chlorpheniramine maleate 1 mg., and phenylephrine hydrochloride 12.5 mg.

Sinutab Tablets (Warner-Chilcott)—Contains acetaminophen 150 mg., phenacetin 150 mg., phenylpropanolamine hydrochloride 25 mg., and phenyltoloxamine citrate 22 mg.

Sinutab II Tablets (Warner-Chilcott)—Contains acetaminophen 150 mg., phenacetin 150 mg., and phenylpropanolamine hydrochloride 25 mg. (Same as Sinutab Tablets but without the antihistamine.)

666 Cold Preparation (Monticello Drug)—Contains phenylpropanolamine hydrochloride, sodium salicylate, epsom salts, ammonium chloride, and sodium citrate.

Triaminicin Tablets (Dorsey)—Contains phenylpropanolamine 25 mg., pheniramine maleate 12.5 mg., pyrilamine maleate 12.5 mg., aspirin 225 mg., acetaminophen 150 mg., caffeine 30 mg., and ascorbic acid 50 mg.

DECONGESTANT NASAL SPRAYS

Alconefrin 25 Nose Drops (Alcon)—Contains phenylephrine hydrochloride 0.25%.

Allerest Nasal Spray (Pharmacraft)—Contains phenylephrine hydrochloride and methapyrilene.

Anahist Decongestant Nasal Spray (Warner-Lambert)—Contains thonzylamine hydrochloride 1% and phenylephrine hydrochloride 0.25%.

Biomydrin Decongestant Nasal Mist (Warner-Chilcott)—Contains phenylephrine hydrochloride 0.25%.

Contac Nasal Mist (Menley & James)—Contains phenylephrine hydrochloride ½% and methapyrilene hydrochloride 0.2%.

Coricidin Decongestant Nasal Mist (Schering)—Contains chlorpheniramine gluconate 3 mg. and phenylephrine hydrochloride 5 mg. (in each 1 cc).

Dristan Decongestant Nasal Mist (Whitehall)—Contains phenylephrine hydrochloride, pheniramine maleate, and benzalkonium chloride.

4-Way Nasal Spray (Bristol-Myers)—Contains phenylephrine hydrochloride, naphazoline hydrochloride, phenylpropanolamine hydrochloride, and pyrilamine maleate.

Mistol Mist (Plough)—Contains phenylephrine hydrochloride 0.25% and methapyrilene fumarate 0.2%.

Nasocon Nasal Spray (Smith, Miller, Patch)—Contains antazoline 0.5% and naphazoline hydrochloride 0.025%.

Neo-Synephrine Nasal Spray (Winthrop)—Contains phenylephrine hydrochloride 0.25% and 0.50%.

Neo-Synephrine Nose Drops (Winthrop)—Contains phenylephrine hydrochloride 1%.

Privine Nasal Spray (Ciba)—Contains naphazoline hydrochloride 0.05%. (Also Nose Drops, the same 0.05%.)

Sinex Nasal Spray (Vick)—Contains phenylephrine hydrochloride, methapyrilene hydrochloride, and cetylpyridinium chloride.

Vapex Inhalant (Fougera)—Contains menthol, oils of lavender and eucalyptus, cineol, linalyl acetate, oil of pine, terebene, borneol, and alcohol 69%. (Not a decongestant.)

INHALERS

Benzedrex Inhaler (Smith Kline & French)—Contains propylhexedrine 250 mg. and menthol 12.5 mg.

Dristan Decongestant Inhaler (Whitehall)—Contains propylhexedrine 250 mg.

Vicks Inhaler (Vick)—Contains l-desoxyephedrine, methol, camphor, methyl salicylate, and bromyl acetate.

COUGH OR THROAT LOZENGES

Cepacol Anesthetic Troches (Merrell)—Contains benzocaine and Ceepryn (cetylpyridinium chloride).

Chloraseptic Lozenges (Eaton)—Contains phenol and sodium phenolate (total phenol 32.5 mg.), menthol and thymol.

Lactona Anesthetic Lozenges (Warner-Lambert)—Contains benzocaine.

Listerine Throat Lozenges (Warner-Lambert)—Contains hexachlorophene. Different flavors. Children's contain 2.4 mg. hexachlorophene.

Lozilles Lozenges (White)—Contains propyl-*p*-aminobenzoate (an anesthetic).

Smith Brothers Medicated Cough Drops (Warner-Lambert)—Contains benzocaine, menthol, and eucalyptol.

Spec-T Antibacterial Troches (Squibb)—Contains cetylpyridinium chloride with benzocaine.

Spec-T Decongestant Troches (Squibb)—Contains benzocaine 10 mg., phenylephrine hydrochloride 5 mg., and phenylpropanolamine hydrochloride 10.5 mg.

Sucrets Antiseptic Throat Lozenges (Calgon/Merck)—Contains 2.4 mg. hexylresorcinol.

Sucrets Cold Decongestant Formula Lozenges (Calgon/Merck)—Contains benzocaine, phenylephrine hydrochloride, and phenylpropanolamine hydrochloride.

Sucrets Cough Control Formula Lozenges (Calgon/Merck)—Contains dextromethorphan and benzocaine.

Thantis Lozenges (Hynson, Westcott & Dunning)—Contains merodicein 1/8 gr. (topical antiseptic) and saligenin 1 gr. (topical anesthetic).

Vicks Cough Silencers (Vick)—Contains dextromethorphan, benzocaine, menthol, anethole, and peppermint oil.

Vicks Medicated Cough Drops (Vick)—Contains menthol, thymol, eucalyptus oil, camphor, tolu and benzyl alcohol.

Victors Dual Action Cough Drops (Vick)—Contains menthol and eucalyptus oil.

COUGH PREPARATIONS

Anahist Honey Lemon Plus Liquid (Warner-Lambert)—Contains dextromethorphan and honey.

Arrestin Cough Medicine (Thayer)—Contains dextromethorphan hydrobromide 10 mg., glyceryl guaiacolate 25 mg., sodium citrate 50 mg., chloroform 29.5 mg., and alcohol 10%.

C³ Cold Cough Capsules (Menley & James)—Contains chlorpheniramine maleate 4 mg., phenylpropanolamine hydrochloride 50 mg., and dextromethorphan hydrobromide 30 mg.

Cheracol D Cough Syrup (Upjohn)—Contains (per 1 fld oz.) dextromethorphan hydrobromide 60 mg., glyceryl guaiacolate 1⅖ gr., ammonium chloride 8 gr., antimony and potassium tartrate 1/12 gr., alcohol 3%, and chloroform 2 gr.

Consotuss Syrup (Merrell)—Contains dextromethorphan hydrobromide 15 mg., glyceryl guaiacolate 100 mg., doxylamine succinate 3.75 mg., alcohol 10%, and chloroform 0.5%.

Coricidin Cough Formula Syrup (Schering)—Contains chlorpheniramine maleate 2 mg., phenylpropanolamine hydrochloride 12.5 mg., glyceryl guaiacolate 50 mg., and ammonium chloride 100 mg.

Coryban-D Cough Syrup (Roerig)—Contains chlorpheniramine maleate 1 mg., phenylephrine hydrochloride 5 mg., acetaminophen 120 mg., glyceryl guaiacolate 50 mg., ascorbic acid 12.5 mg., chloroform 0.05%, alcohol 7.5%, and dextromethorphan hydrobromide 7.5 mg.

Cosanyl-DM Cough Syrup (Parke, Davis)—Contains dextromethorphan hydrobromide 15 mg., phenylephrine hydrochloride 5 mg., and alcohol 6%.

Cough Calmers Lozenges (Robins)—Contains dextromethorphan 7.5 mg. and glyceryl guaiacolate 50 mg.

Creomulsion Cough Medicine (Creomulsion Co.)—Contains beechwood creosote, cascara, ipecac, menthol, white pine, wild cherry, and alcohol 1%.

Creo-Terpin Compound (Denver)—Contains terpin hydrate 2 gr., creosote 2 min., sodium glycerophosphate 4 gr., and alcohol 25%.

Dondril Tablets (Whitehall)—Contains dextromethorphan hydrobromide 10 mg., phenylephrine hydrochloride 5 mg., chlorpheniramine maleate 1 mg., and glyceryl guaiacolate 50 mg.

Dristan Decongestant [Liquid] (Whitehall)—Contains dextromethorphan hydrobromide 7.5 mg., phenylephrine hydrochloride 5 mg., chlorpheniramine maleate 1 mg., sodium citrate, glyceryl guaiacolate, chloroform, and alcohol 12%.

Father John's Medicine for Coughs & Colds (Father John's)—Contains cod liver oil, gum arabic, and glycerine (a cod liver oil emulsion).

Novahistine Elixir (Dow)—Contains phenylephrine hydrochloride 5 mg., chlorpheniramine maleate 1 mg., chloroform, and alcohol 5%.

NyQuil Liquid (Vick)—Contains acetaminophen 600 mg./fld oz., ephedrine sulfate, doxylamine succinate, dextromethorphan hydrobromide, and alcohol 25%.

Pertussin 8-Hour Cough Formula (Chesebrough-Pond's)—Contains dextromethorphan hydrobromide, sodium citrate, ammonium chloride, chloroform 0.3%, and alcohol 9.5% by volume.

Pertussin Plus (Chesebrough-Pond's)—Contains acetaminophen, dextromethorphan hydrobromide, phenylephrine hydrochloride, chlorpheniramine maleate, and alcohol 25%.

Pertussin Wild Berry Cough Syrup (Chesebrough-Pond's)—Contains dextromethorphan hydrobromide, sodium citrate, ammonium chloride, alcohol 8.5%, and chloroform 0.2%.

Pinex Concentrate (Pinex Co.)—Contains oil of pine tar, potassium guaiacol sulfonate, oil of eucalyptus, extract grindelia, glycerine, chloroform 18 min., and alcohol 17%. (Directions call for dilution with syrup.)

Pinex Cough Syrup (Pinex Co.)—Contains potassium guaiacol sulfonate, oil of pine tar, eucalyptus oil, extract grindelia, glycerine, alcohol 3%, and chloroform 3 min.

Rem Cough Medicine (Block Drug)—Contains squill, ipecac, lobelia, wild cherry, blood root, horehound, white pine, tar, tolu, menthol, glycerine, ammonium chloride, alcohol 1.2%, chloroform 0.7%, and benzyl alcohol 0.2%.

Robitussin-DM 6–8 Hour Cough Formula (Robins)—Contains glyceryl guaiacolate 100 mg., dextromethorphan hydrobromide 15 mg., and alcohol 1.4%.

Romilar Cough Discs (Sauter/Hoffmann-LaRoche)—Contains dextromethorphan hydrobromide and benzyl alcohol.

Romilar CF 8-Hour Cough Formula (Sauter/Hoffmann-LaRoche)—Contains dextromethorphan hydrobromide, chlorpheniramine maleate, acetaminophen, ipecac, chloroform 0.25%, and alcohol 10%.

Spec-T Cough Suppressant Troches (Squibb)—Contains benzocaine 10 mg. and dextromethorphan hydrobromide 10 mg.

Trind-DM Expectorant (Mead Johnson)—Contains phenylephrine hydrochloride 2.5 mg., acetaminophen 150 mg., dextromethorphan hydrobromide 7.5 mg., glyceryl guaiacolate 50 mg., and alcohol 15%.

Vicks Cough Syrup (Vick)—Contains dextromethorphan hydrobromide, glyceryl guaiacolate, sodium citrate, chloroform, and alcohol 5%.

Vicks Formula 44 Extra Strength Cough Discs (Vick)—Contains dextromethorphan and benzocaine.

Vicks Formula 44 Extra Strength Cough Mixture (Vick)—Contains dextromethorphan hydrobromide, doxylamine succinate, sodium citrate, chloroform, and alcohol 10%. (The "extra strength" presumably resides in the doxylamine—compare with Vicks Cough Syrup.)

MEDICATED ROOM VAPORIZERS

Congestaid Aersosol Medication (Colgate-Palmolive)—Contains camphor, eucalyptol, thymol, menthol, triethylene and dipropylene glycol, and alcohol 17%.

Dristan Medicated Room Vaporizer (Whitehall)—Contains camphor, menthol, eucalyptol, dipropylene glycol, triethylene glycol, and alcohol 17%.

Kaz Mist—Medicated Aerosol (Kaz Mfg.)—Contains dipropylene glycol, menthol, camphor, oil of eucalyptus, oil of peppermint, oil of lavender, and methyl salicylate.

Pertussin Medicated Vaporizer (Chesebrough-Pond's)—Contains triethylene glycol, dipropylene glycol, menthol, and eucalyptol.

VapoSteam Liquid Medication for Hot Steam Vaporizers (Vick)—Contains polyoxyethylene dodecanol, menthol, camphor, eucalyptus oil, tincture of benzoin, and alcohol 55%. To be poured directly into water in hot steam vaporizer or bowl.

DRUGS FOR CHILDREN

Children are not little adults from the standpoint of disease. They differ in many aspects: first, a psychological assault can have much more profound and lasting damage than a comparable one in adults; second, they are subject to diseases somewhat different—often in kind as well as in degree—from those in adults. And the impact of disease on children also differs.

The premonitory signs of an oncoming illness may have only a minor symptom—e.g., no appetite. Do not push a meal into an unwilling child. Be aware and alert for any other deviations. A child may be coming down with an infection.

Children are much more sensitive to certain imbalances in the body and more responsive to them. Their recovery rate also differs; a younger person tends to "bounce back" more quickly and perhaps with less physical damage.

For these and other reasons, giving young children fractions of adult doses, except in the simplest of conditions, is not treating children safely and adequately.

For example, one facet in drug administration that we take for granted, in adults as well as in children, is the dose. This is a troublesome problem. No one dose is the optimum; doses are average doses and the average may not apply best to each individual. (The published doses in the official compendia are more legal than medical; in the USP they are only the dose from which to start. Ideally, the dose should be modified upward or downward by the physician, to obtain that amount which will give maximal response with a minimum of side effects.)

As with any drug—and this is especially important in children—the question always arises of not only what drug to give but how much of it to give. The dose is as significant a consideration as the choice of the drug itself.

There are several rules for determining children's dosages, all of which leave something to be desired. One rule is based on weight; another is based on age; an additional one is based on the size of the child calculated on body area, which is perhaps the most desirable but requires calculation before prescribing. But unfortunately all of them are derived from the adult dose.

Another point of importance regarding the dose: medicine is given to children when they are sick. And it is just when sick that they may not be able to tolerate a given drug which otherwise they could. For example, they can tolerate aspirin for a cold, but when they have a stomach upset they may not be able to tolerate it or tolerate it as well.

We make these points to emphasize the importance of drugs and their dosages in children—and why one should not casually consider that just less of an adult dose is fine for children.

These are basic to our belief that one cannot put reliance on treating children casually. This is the reason why we are not supplying a comprehensive listing of children's drugs, except those found at the end of this chapter. But remember that "half-doses" isn't a safe and effective rule.

Yet there are certain drugs that can be used for children under certain conditions. However, the time of expected response should be shortened. For example, with analgesics, adults are cautioned that if no improvement with self-medication occurs within one to two weeks, a physician should be consulted. But if no improvement occurs within a few days when you are giving a child an over-the-counter drug available without prescription, the child should be taken to a physician. Even if the physician, after examining the child, advises the mother to continue giving the aspirin or other drug she may have administered, there is an advantage in knowing that nothing more serious, requiring other measures, has been found. And one cannot tell in advance.

For fever in children, aspirin is still the most desirable remedy, though it is merely treating the symptom. The so-called children's aspirin, containing 1¼ gr. of aspirin per tablet, is ¼ the strength of regular aspirin tablets. They are a convenient form of administration in that they prevent the need of breaking tablets to administer the dose. Moreover, they are usually flavored and probably can be administered with less resistance on the part of the child. The usual dose for a 3- or 4-year-old child is one tablet of the *children's* aspirin; two such tablets for a 4- to 5-year-old child; three such tablets for a 6- to 8-year-old child, four such tablets (or one regular adult aspirin tablet) for a 9-year-old child or older.

Another rule of thumb for aspirin—but one in which the dosage is higher than just stated—is 1 grain of aspirin per year of age up to 10 years of age.

The single dose of acetaminophen differs: in children 1 year old give 1 grain; 2 to 3 years old, 1½ grains; 3 to 6 years old, 1½ to 2 grains; 6 to 12 years old, 3 to 4 grains. These too are approximations. The dose for salicylamide is somewhat smaller. When using these products instead of—*not in addition to*—aspirin follow the detailed dose schedule on the labels. All good brands are comparable, and one is as reliable or as deficient as another.

In many drugs, though there are notable exceptions, the lower level of an adult dose is given to children 12 to 14 years old, and regular adult doses over 14 years old.

Cough mixtures or antidiarrheal drugs may be given to children, but only those adult preparations that carry a dosage for children should be used. However, diarrhea may be a serious situation in children, as in a short time diarrhea may produce loss of essential salts and water, and can dehydrate a child more quickly than an adult.

Severe diarrhea in an infant or young child *can be fatal* in one or two days. If the child is not vomiting and can take fluids, the diarrhea is less worrisome. If the child is vomiting and has diarrhea, a physician should be called the same day.

More poisoning is reported in children than in any other age group. Children 1 to 4 years old account for 63% of poisonings reported in the United States. For that reason, two items should be in the medicine chest of any household that has children. One is syrup of ipecac; the other is powdered activated charcoal.

But we *do not* mean to imply that poisoning can be treated at home. The *first* thing to do in poisoning is to call a doctor. Then, if he tells you to use ipecac or charcoal until he arrives, you should have it on hand.

Syrup of ipecac induces vomiting. It is available in most drugstores, and a ready-packed variety containing two doses, where no spoon or other measuring device is necessary, can be obtained. For that reason it is preferable.

While the stomach tube is often used to wash poisonous ingredients out of the stomach, it is not used in the event of poisoning by corrosives—such as lye, or oils, or petroleum products such as insecticides. This does *not* mean that ipecac can be used in these cases. In some cases of poisoning, as by corrosives, a stomach tube can perforate the stomach. Vomiting can further damage the foodpipe by regurgitation. (Corrosives are neutralized in the stomach.)

The other product, powdered activated charcoal, does not induce vomiting, and is often given after vomiting. The reason for its administration is to pick up—adsorb—any remaining poison in the stomach. It is given by mixing thoroughly 2 teaspoonfuls (10 grams) powdered charcoal with about ¼ glass of water, and having the child quickly drink the slurry.

Salt is recommended in some first aid manuals as an emetic, to induce vomiting in poisoning. Don't use it! There is a considerable hazard connected with its use, especially in children, by gravely disturbing their body equilibrium of chloride and sodium. While occasionally successful in inducing vomiting it can create formidable problems, especially in children, and more particularly when a child has taken a poison. Salt is a poison in its own right when taken in more than the quantities customarily used in food.

To search for or to run to buy a preparation to combat poisoning when it is needed is too late! These products should be prominently located in the medicine chest, and adults should familiarize themselves with their use *before* they are needed. Did you ever try to read, understand and implement directions when you are hit by an emergency?

But above all, in poisoning, first call your doctor.

NAMES OF PRODUCTS

FOR POISONING

Powdered Activated Charcoal (Requa)—Do not use tablets for poisoning—only powder. The virtue of the powder resides in the great surface exposed by powder particles, which adsorb poisons.

Syrup of Ipecac (Alliance)—Consists of syrup of ipecac with a package insert that clearly conveys the method of use.

FOR TREATMENT OF SYMPTOMS OF THE COLD

Aspirin for Children (St. Joseph, Bayer, etc.)—Each tablet contains 1¼ grains aspirin, usually orange-flavored. (Analgesic and antipyretic [fever reducing].)

Biact Tablets (Sauter/Hoffmann-LaRoche)—Contains aspirin 1¼ grains, phenylephrine hydrochloride 6¼ mg. (Decongestant.)

Children's Bufferin (Bristol-Myers)—Contains aspirin 1¼ grains with aluminum magnesium buffers. (Analgesic and antipyretic.)

Children's Romilar Cough Syrup (Sauter/Hoffmann-LaRoche)—Contains dextromethorphan hydrobromide 7.5 mg., glyceryl guaiacolate 25 mg., with sodium citrate and citric acid. (Cough suppressant.)

Coricidin Demilets Tablets (Schering)—Contains chlorpheniramine maleate 0.5 mg.. phenylephrine 2.5 mg., and aspirin 80 mg. (Decongestant.)

Coricidin Medilets Tablets, Cold Relief for Children (Schering)—Contains Chlor-Trimeton 0.5 mg. and aspirin 1¼ grains. (Analgesic and antipyretic.)

Liquiprin (Thayer)—Contains 1 mg. salicylamide per 1 cc (5 mg. per teaspoonful). (Analgesic and antipyretic.)

Romilar Chewable Cough Tablets for Children (Sauter/Hoffmann-LaRoche)—Contains 7.5 mg. dextromethorphan hydrobromide and 2.0 mg. benzocaine. (Cough suppressant.)

St. Joseph Cough Syrup for Children (Plough)—Contains 7.5 mg. dextromethorphan. (Cough suppressant.)

St. Joseph Liquid "A" (Plough)—Children's analgesic drops. Contains acetaminophen.

Valadol Chewable Tablets (Squibb)—Contains acetaminophen 120 mg. (2 gr.).

Valadol Liquid (Squibb)—Contains acetaminophen 120 mg. (2 gr.).

CHEST RUBS

Mentholatum (Mentholatum)—Contains menthol, camphor, boric acid, and aromatic oils in petrolatum base.

Musterole (Plough)—Contains volatile oil of mustard, camphor, menthol, and synthetic oil of wintergreen.

Penetro Analgesic Rub (Plough)—Contains methyl salicylate, turpentine, menthol, camphor, thymol, and pine oil in mutton suet base.

VapoRub (Vick)—Contains camphor, menthol, spirits of turpentine, eucalyptus oil, cedar leaf oil, nutmeg oil, and thymol.

FOR DIARRHEA

Kaopectate (Upjohn)—Contains kaolin 90 mg. and pectin 130 mg.

STOMACH AND ABDOMINAL DISCOMFORTS

STOMACH UPSET AND ANTACIDS

DEFINITION

Stomach or abdominal discomfort can take many forms. One may be a burning sensation called heartburn, sour stomach or hyperacidity, a pain in the pit of the stomach, i.e., the upper abdomen, which is usually referred to as indigestion, belching and gas. It is a general feeling which is lumped under the phrase "upset stomach."

CAUSE

There are numerous causes for this type of discomfort, some of which can be serious. But frequently, when it casually occurs, it may be due to nervous tension, eating too much, eating too rapidly, or eating a food that may disagree with a given individual. Cucumbers, for example, can affect some or garlic others. The eating of food mixtures is usually not the cause of discomfort; for example, pickles and ice cream will not upset you provided that you tolerate pickles or have no intolerance to fats such as ice cream. Reports of food incompatibilities are usually myths.

DISCUSSION AND CAUTIONS

Every incident of indigestion is surely not a heart attack, but you should be aware of the fact that a moderate spell of indigestion can sometimes be a sign of a heart attack.

Occasionally, the pain of a heart attack will mimic indigestion. If pain occurs on the left side of the lower chest or in the center or pit of the stomach (epigastric pain), with no feeling of burning, and if it is persistent and is not shortly alleviated by antacids, your physician should be called. This is especially true if you previously had heart trouble, and if you are a man over 35 or 40 years old.

Similarly, heartburn or similar stomach symptoms may be due to a hiatus hernia. A hiatus hernia is a break or herniation of a portion of the upper stomach through the diaphragm into the chest. This is a common condition in people over 50 years old, and frequently no symptoms appear. However, in some people it allows the stomach acid to wash upon the lower food pipe, or esophagus, and cause a burning pain.

There are to be sure other conditions that may cause stomach or abdominal discomfort so, if pain persists, do not attempt self-diagnosis but call your doctor.

INGREDIENTS

Antacids are used for those conditions that are lumped together as heartburn, sour stomach, hyperacidity, etc. The reason for their use is that they neutralize stomach acidity; nearly all of them are mildly alkaline.

Among antacids, the commonly used ones are aluminum hydroxide, calcium carbonate (chalk), magnesium trisilicate, magnesium hydroxide, magnesium carbonate, and sodium bicarbonate (baking soda).

The magnesium salts—hydroxide, carbonate, and also trisilicate—tend to be laxative. Aluminum hydroxide is a good antacid but often constipating. For that reason most antacids contain both aluminum and magnesium salts. Magnesium salts do not constipate. Magnesium hydroxide is the common milk of magnesia.

Sodium bicarbonate is an effective and quickly acting antacid, but its antacid effect is quickly dissipated. There is also a likelihood of alkalosis—a turning of the reaction of the blood to slightly increased alkalinity—if too much is used or if it is used too frequently. Also, extra sodium from sodium bicarbonate may not be desirable for people who have high blood pressure or a heart condition, as the extra sodium may cause further high blood pressure or even edema—an accumulation of fluid in the tissues.

A good antacid will therefore contain both aluminum hydroxide and one of the magnesium salts. It is improved when calcium carbonate or chalk is added, as it is somewhat more persistent, and is less likely than aluminum hydroxide to cause constipation, and its carbonate portion reacts with acid.

These insoluble ingredients—namely, hydroxide, trisilicate, carbonate of magnesium, or aluminum hydroxide, all of which are insoluble in water but are suspended in water in the liquid antacids—neutralize acidity and are believed to soothe the irritated mucous membrane of the stomach. Hence, they increase comfort, often relieve the individual and allow him to belch up entrapped gas. The latter case is especially true of effervescent products. (Note: the stomach fluids are normally slightly acid; if neutralized they soon redevelop acidity, which is normal, but in the meantime the individual is relieved.)

Antacids are available in liquid, tablet, and powder forms. If taken in the form of tablets, the tablets should be thoroughly chewed, not swallowed whole. The principal point is to have the ingredients of the tablets in as fine a subdivision as possible so that when swallowed, they have a greater area to neutralize stomach acid faster. For that reason liquids are preferred, but powders, well mixed with water, are equally useful. Tablets are the third choice because their spreadability is not as great even when well chewed and swallowed. However, tablets are convenient to carry and it is vastly better to carry and use tablets during the day than not use them at all when needed. The active ingredients are intended to, and do, adsorb acid and neutralize acidity.

Antacids with an antispasmodic such as belladonna, or sedatives such as barbiturates, are available only on prescription. These products are more particularly used in peptic ulcer, colitis, or other abdominal conditions. Other antacids also contain a silicone ingredient, simethicone, which breaks up the bubbles of entrapped gas, allowing for its expulsion by belching. Antacids containing simethicone are particularly used when flatulence (gas) is present.

One antacid, Kolantyl, available both as a liquid as well as wafer, contains an ingredient which represses acid formation. That ingredient (Bentyl) is referred to as an anticholinergic —i.e., it works through the nervous system and reduces the secretion of acid. It also reduces other secretions; hence, as a side effect, it may cause dryness of the mouth. But that side effect is a small price to pay for the relief from stomach discomfort.

Effervescent tablets containing aspirin raise a point. Should aspirin be taken during a stomach upset? Aspirin irritates the stomach and in a small but significant proportion of people produces bleeding. Therefore we are wary about its use in connection with stomach discomfort.

However, the aspirin in effervescent tablets is converted into sodium acetyl salicylate (sodium aspirin) when in solution, with sodium bicarbonate. The sodium derivative of aspirin is not acid and has not been reported to cause the bleeding known to take place with aspirin. Its judicious use should not present dangers.

A few antacids also contain a small amount of digestive enzymes, with the idea that they help the digestive process. Whether enzymes given by mouth are helpful, as contrasted with those elaborated in the body in the normal process of digestion, is a point on which there are clearly divided opinions. Some feel that they are useless.

In case of failure of kidney function or phosphorus depletion, no aluminum antacid should be used.

We have often reflected how unpredictable taste can be. One of us, for example, hates the taste of wintergreen. If you find that, say, Zilch's tablets are highly recommended but have a flavor that virtually turns your stomach, don't take them. Otherwise, you may come away with a worse stomach upset than you set out to correct.

If Your Need Is for a Product Against Stomach and Abdominal Discomfort (Acid or Upset Stomach or Heartburn):

Look for Products Containing the Following Ingredients:

- Calcium carbonate (chalk)
- Aluminum hydroxide
- Magnesium trisilicate
- Magnesium carbonate
- Magnesium hydroxide
- Activated charcoal
- Simethicone
- Papain

Avoid the Following Ingredients:

- Sodium bicarbonate or baking soda (preferably avoided)

NAMES OF PRODUCTS

Al-Caroid Antacid Powder (Breon)—Contains calcium carbonate, aluminum hydroxide, magnesium hydroxide, and papain. Papain is a protein-digesting enzyme.

Alka-Seltzer (Miles)—Contains sodium bicarbonate, citric acid, aspirin, and a calcium phosphate. Tablets only, which effervesce when dropped in water—and must be taken only in water. While it neutralizes acidity, it does not have the protective and coating effect of the aluminum-calcium-magnesium antacids. However, the gas (carbon dioxide) released upon effervescence may bring up entrapped gas. Also, the aspirin present (5 gr. per tablet), in the form of sodium acetyl salicylate, may be advantageous in associated headache or symptoms of the common cold. Contains a small amount of sodium from solution of the sodium bicarbonate.

Amphojel (Wyeth)—Contains only aluminum hydroxide. Liquid and tablets.

Bisodol (American Home)—Contains magnesium trisilicate, magnesium hydroxide, and calcium carbonate. Less likely to constipate as it contains no aluminum hydroxide. Calcium carbonate as an ingredient is an advantage in an antacid. Powder and tablets.

Brioschi Seltzer (Brioschi, Inc.)—Contains sodium bicarbonate and tartaric acid. Similar to Eno Sparkling Antacid and Alka-Seltzer but contains no aspirin.

Camalox Suspension (Rorer)—Contains magnesium and aluminum hydroxides and calcium carbonate. Similar to Maalox but has the advantage of containing calcium carbonate. Liquid and tablets.

Charcoal Tablets (Requa)—Consists of wood charcoal. While not an antacid it is used often for expelling gas or adsorbing breakdown products of foods that may cause discomfort. This is based on the old and still viable premise of charcoal as an *ad*sorbing agent in poisoning. It may immobilize poisons in the intestinal tract but it has no effect on poisons already *ab*sorbed into the bloodstream. When taking the tablets chew them well and swallow with water. The more effective—and also the more messy—way is to take charcoal powder, because then adsorption is at optimum.

Cremalin (Winthrop)—Contains aluminum hydroxide and magnesium hydroxide. Liquid and tablets.

Delcid Suspension (Merrell)—Contains aluminum hydroxide and magnesium hydroxide.

Ducon Antacid (Smith Kline & French)—Contains aluminum hydroxide, magnesium hydroxide, and calcium carbonate. Liquid only.

Eno Sparkling Antacid (Beecham)—Contains sodium bicarbonate and sodium tartrate. Similar to Alka-Seltzer but contains no aspirin.

Gelusil (Warner-Chilcott)—Contains magnesium trisilicate and aluminum hydroxide. Liquid and tablets. (Also available as Gelusil M tablets containing mannitol.)

Kolantyl (Merrell)—Contains Bentyl (dicyclomine hydrochloride), aluminum hydroxide, magnesium hydroxide, and methyl cellulose. Bentyl belongs to a group of substances called anticholinergics, which reduce stomach acidity, a desirable step in duodenal ulcer treatment. Kolantyl is an effective antacid as well, due to the presence of other ingredients. Methyl cellulose is merely a demulcent. Liquid and wafers.

Maalox (Rorer)—Contains magnesium and aluminum hydroxide in a colloidal suspension. In form of liquid and tablets, single and double strength tablets.

Milk of Magnesia (Various Manufacturers)—Consists of magnesium hydroxide, a laxative as well as an antacid. Of advantage as an antacid to older people who are frequently constipated. Should be taken in a glassful of water for best effect. The liquid is distinctly better than tablets.

Mylanta (Stuart)—Contains aluminum hydroxide and magnesium hydroxide and simethicone, a silicone product. Liquid and tablets.

Pepto-Bismol (Norwich)—The liquid contains bismuth subsalicylate, salol, and zinc phenolsulfonate in a demulcent base. The bismuth salt is protective and coating. The salol and zinc phenolsulfonate are mildly antiseptic and claimed to be useful for this purpose. The tablets contain bismuth subsalicylate, calcium carbonate, glycocol (aminoacetic acid). More particularly an antacid as compared to the liquid. Liquid and tablets.

Riopan (Ayerst)—Contains magnesium and aluminum hydroxides said to have a buffering action. Liquid and tablets.

Seidlitz Powder (Various Manufacturers)—Consists of powder in blue packages and white packages; one blue and one white paper making a set. Blue paper contains sodium bicarbonate and potassium and sodium tartrate; white paper contains tartaric acid. The contents of a blue and a white paper are dissolved separately, then mixed, and taken after effervescence has somewhat reduced. Similar to Alka-Seltzer, but contains no aspirin. Contains sodium, as all effervescent products do, and therefore people who must restrict their sodium intake should take it only with care, if at all.

Silain-Gel (Plough)—Similar to Mylanta.

Tums (Lewis-Howe)—Contains calcium carbonate, magnesium carbonate, magnesium trisilicate, and sodium bicarbonate. Contains a very small amount of sodium per tablet (3 mg. or less) from sodium bicarbonate; hence people with salt-restricted diets should be aware of its contents.

Win-Gel (Winthrop)—Contains aluminum-magnesium hydroxides. Liquid and tablets.

CONSTIPATION AND LAXATIVES

DEFINITION

It is difficult to define constipation because normally there is no set frequency of defecation. It varies from person to person, and "averages" would be meaningless. It must be compared with the individual's previous pattern or history of passing stool. It cannot be defined by frequency. Nor can constipation be defined by the hardness, dryness, or difficulty of passing stool.

But by and large, probably most people pass stools anywhere from daily up to as infrequently as once every 3 or 4 days. Habit, among other factors, plays a great part in the frequency of stool passing. The term *obstipation* is the same as constipation but usually connotes a more severe form. The term *costive* (adj.) means merely *constipated.*

CAUSE

We shall concern ourselves mainly with simple constipation (rectal constipation). It is usually due to a weak nervous defecating reflex or an accumulation of dried and often semi-impacted stool in the rectum. (Marked impaction of stool in the rectum requires manual removal which is done professionally.) The accumulation of stool in the rectum—where it loses its fluid component and becomes hard—often is due to a voluntary delay in moving bowels.

Constipation and stool accumulation can also be caused by (a) a change in activity such as bed rest or other inactivity; (b) travel during which one's routine, hence habit patterns are changed; (c) change in the diet to one having less roughage or fluid than customary; or (d) emotional upset. A relatively *sudden* onset of constipation may be due to the above causes, but a change in bowel habits may possibly have graver reasons. Among the latter may be cancer of the rectum in which there is a progressive constipation and a decrease in the caliber or thickness of the stool. Constipation alternating with diarrhea may be due to spastic colon as well as a tumor in the intestines. Other causes may be vascular, as in the case of stroke, or psychological as in depression or severe neurosis or psychosis. Additional causes include tuberculosis and hypothyroidism. Certain drugs, particularly sedatives, codeine, aluminum hydroxide or calcium used as antacids, are other causes of constipation.

Usually, a sudden onset of constipation suggests that there may be something wrong with one of the body mechanisms involved in the act of defecation, such as muscular, in which the nervous impulses controlling contractions are weak, probably triggered by a reduction of nervous reflexes. Recently, a new view of the possible origin of constipation was offered—a hereditary factor. The mechanism is believed to be a hereditary tendency of the bowel to absorb too much water, resulting in hard stools.

DISCUSSION AND CAUTIONS

Probably more instances of constipation are caused by behavioral rather than physiological reasons.

There are several reasons for the behavioral or psychological causes: (a) bowel movements are highly sensitive to timing, and if no daily pattern has been established, and observed routinely, the frequency of passing stool will be erratic; (b) the acts relating to the passing of stool are involved with a number of atavistic beliefs, hence external and cultural factors affect it; (c) a bowel movement is considered to be an act of purification, hence the almost automatic recourse to laxatives; and (d) stool has a negative connotation in the social framework. For example, when visiting, an individual is perhaps reluctant to excuse himself and enter the toilet for a bowel movement if he has an alternative. He has an alternative: he can usually resist and suppress his urge with little discomfort, hence delay it, allowing stool to accumulate and harden, which will be passed later with more difficulty.

To cause bowel evacuation or make the movement less stressful, any of a group of products are used, known collectively as laxatives. Laxatives facilitate evacuation, render stools fluid or softer, and give a feeling of "relief" from distention and other discomfort when stools accumulate.

The term *cathartic* is the same as laxative, except that a cathartic may connote an agent that produces a more energetic action than a laxative. But words are invested with meanings due to their usage, over and above what they may actually denote. A *purgative* is a more energetic agent than a cathartic. The word *purge* has a long history (purification) and is used in various disciplines; for example in law, purge of contempt, and in theology, purge of heresy, purge of sin, etc. The term *physic,* which has an ancient history, means a laxative without the emotional overtones that *purge* confers. The origin of the word *cathartic* is related to *clean;* that of laxative is related to *loose* (laxation).

Thus people often take laxatives for atavistic and psychological reasons, depending on the culture in which they live. For example, at the beginning of the twentieth century, and for about 20 to 40 years thereafter, it was customary in many parts of the United States for most of the family to take a *physic* on Saturday night. The choice of Saturday evening was probably dictated by the fact that Sunday was not a working day. But nowhere is it explained how the urge to defecate simultaneously was served for several members of a family that had only one toilet, and often had to share even that with neighbors.

People in the Middle Ages were bled and purged as a remedy for a variety of ills. Many of our contemporaries continue to purge themselves. The frequency varies. Yet, in response to a learned habit, people believe that aiding the expulsion of stool by laxation confers a greater good than unassisted movement alone. They believe that laxation purifies, relieves headache, dusts cobwebs from brains, and improves the condition of the skin. While severe constipation (if not due to graver causes such as tuberculosis, hypothyroidism, etc.) may cause headache and loss of appetite, there is no good reason for the regular taking of laxatives except, perhaps, among the aged, many of whom tend to move bowels with some difficulty, especially if they are inactive. While laxatives do not contain habituating drugs, the *regular practice* of taking laxatives is habit-forming; it does not allow the body to establish its own habit, i.e., a pattern of bowel movements, by timing and diet.

With older people, their muscular tone is low, their reflexes are commonly sluggish, and their constipation often leads to the impaction of stool in the rectum. Some cannot tolerate roughage; if they markedly increase their fluid intake they may overload their circulation–many of them live with some tolerable degree of congestive heart failure which is kept under some degree of compensation. Laxatives, carefully chosen to fit the individual need of these people, are the alternative to periods of constipation followed by those of diarrhea due to taking laxatives.

While the habit of regularly taking laxatives is undesirable, it is as bad, or perhaps worse at certain times, to strain at stool. When straining to move bowels, often dried and hardened by storage in the sigmoid (the upper part of the rectum), you perform a maneuver that includes a "bearing-down" or squeezing, with the top of larynx (glottis) closed. This is called the Valsalva maneuver, after an Italian anatomist of the seventeenth century. This chain of events increases pressure within the chest and may lead to stroke, or at least it may increase an already high blood pressure. People with heart disease should avoid straining. Straining at stool also aggravates an existing hernia, or it may open a recent surgical wound of the abdomen. Straining to move bowels has been described as again detaching the retina after an operation for repairing a detached retina.

Therefore, straining at stool should be avoided. To prevent

it a laxative is indeed indicated (1) to soften stool and (2) to increase peristaltic waves. Softening stool alone is often not enough in the event of a reduced muscular tone of the intestine that does not efficiently send its contents along the way for conversion to stool and expulsion. Therefore laxatives that increase peristalsis may be necessary. Of course, the opposite also happens frequently—an overactive muscle tone due to spastic colon.

Another of the events in older people that may add to constipation is depression. Excitement, particularly fear, increases peristaltic waves and a strong urge to pass stool. Diarrhea results. Most animals also defecate instantly when frightened. The contrary is the case in a depression of the emotional tone. There is a reduction in the amplitude of the affects and in a variety of metabolic functions. In fact, many instances of impotence arise from depression. Excitement speeds up peristalsis and depression slows it down. Although it is well known, it is often forgotten that older people, especially those who are retired from active life, have varying degrees of depression. Constipation, in addition to other complaints, has a part in the roots of their depression.

Older people are often preoccupied with bowel movement, and sometimes rightly so. In these instances, unless the nutritional status can be improved—and it often needs improvement—well-chosen laxatives may indeed be indicated. This is not to be understood that we are endorsing a laxative habit. Our point is that it is better to take a well-chosen laxative than to be preoccupied with constipation, especially when you have time for such preoccupation in retirement.

Laxatives as a class are divided into several groups, each group exerting its effect by a different mechanism and, conceivably, to serve different laxative needs.

There are other occasions when a laxative may be advisable. For example, a codeine-containing cough mixture will constipate; or when antacids, which are frequently recommended by a physician, are taken for an extended period of time they may, and usually do, constipate.

In constipation due to the codeine-containing cough mixtures, a stimulant laxative containing acetphenolisatin, senna derivative, or danthron may be preferable because it stimulates peristalsis. In the case of aluminum-containing antacids, which are astringent and drying, bulk laxatives taken with sufficient water are better, for in that case lubrication is usually sufficient to establish bowel movement.

STIMULANT LAXATIVES

Stimulation is merely a matter of degree of irritation (which is a more vigorous stimulation). This group stimulates muscle or nerve junctions to favor peristalsis, creating peristaltic waves to move intestinal contents downward. The stronger the laxation the more griping. Both the intensity and rapidity of effect are a function of the dose.

But this does not mean that a given dose has the same effect in all individuals. The optimum dose that causes adequate, but not excessive, laxation has to be found empirically for each individual, within a reasonably moderate range. The following are members of this group of laxatives:

Phenolphthalein (white and yellow—yellow is more active)
Castor oil
Cascara
Aloin
Senna and its active derivatives
Rhubarb
Danthron (1-8-dihydroxyanthraquinone)
Acetphenolisatin (oxyphenisatin; diacetyldiphenolisatin)
Bisacodyl (active rectally as well as orally)
Casanthranol—similar to senna or cascara group

Castor oil is the most rapid-acting of the group and is effective in about 3 to 4 hours; the others are usually effective in 8 to 24 hours. Stimulant laxatives, except castor oil, are often preferable in older people, as well as for occasional use in others, due to the fact that they stimulate the peristaltic tone of the intestine favoring expulsion. Together with fluid, they make rather loose, often watery stools. While they are reliable in their action, their irritating effect may be undesirable if it is so great as to induce laxation for more than one day or cause three stools during that day.

Phenolphthalein may cause a skin rash in a small percentage of users. But it has been used for decades, and is by and large nontoxic. The only other drawback is on the rare occasions that its laxative action continues for several days.

Within recent years, laxatives containing either bisacodyl, danthron, or acetphenolisatin have become popular. Their effect is exerted within 6 to 12 hours, depending on dose and individual response. Most preparations containing one of the above, are combined with dioctyl sodium sulfosuccinate, which is a wetting agent, hence softens stool, without drawing a great deal of water into the intestine. Two or three soft, but not watery stools may be expected from these combinations. They are rightly favored for use in older people, who need a stimulant to peristaltic action.

A few reports have appeared recently giving data on a total of about a dozen instances of jaundice, ascribed to the use of oxyphenisatin as a laxative. While there is nothing conclusive in establishing the cause and effect relationship, these reports wisely recommend that laxatives containing oxyphenisatin should not be used regularly. For the occasional use, and laxatives should be used only if necessary and occasionally, there is little or no imminent danger. As we go to press an announcement by the FDA proposes to withdraw from the market products containing oxyphenisatin.

LUBRICANT LAXATIVES

This group comprises (a) mineral oil and (b) dioctyl sodium sulfosuccinate. Mineral oil is not absorbed by the gut and is truly a lubricant. When mixed with intestinal contents it softens them, then envelops the stool in an oily coat, facilitating its expulsion due to its lubricity. But plain mineral oil is hardly recommended for use, as it interferes with food absorption in the intestine and may "leak" through at the anus. If lubrication *is* necessary, a mineral oil emulsion of agar, chondrus (Irish moss), or psyllium (see *Bulk Laxatives*) is preferable because the mineral oil is emulsified and less persistent on the intestinal wall. If stimulation of peristalsis is desirable, mineral oil is certainly not the preferable substance, as it does not stimulate peristalsis. The light mineral oil tends to leak through the anus more easily than the heavy mineral oil. The heavy mineral oil is more persistent in coating the intestine and interferes with food absorption for a somewhat longer time.

The most popular form of mineral oil preparations are the mineral oil emulsions with agar. But the amount of gum (agar or even chondrus) is relatively small. The laxative effect is usually fortified by the presence of phenolphthalein.

Dioctyl sodium sulfosuccinate (DOSS) is not an oil, and strictly it is not a lubricant. But it is a wetting agent (similar to detergents), enabling water in the gut to mix with intestinal contents and to soften them, facilitating expulsion. DOSS does not stimulate peristalsis, though combinations of DOSS with stimulant laxatives are available. If softening only is required, DOSS is certainly preferable to mineral oil to help expulsion of intestinal contents. But if DOSS is taken, several glasses of water should be drunk during the day, so that there is enough water present in the gut to be mixed with the intestinal contents.

BULK-FORMING LAXATIVES

One of the stimuli to which the intestine responds with the urge to pass stool is sheer mass. Hence, when the gut is filled with water (see also *Saline Laxatives*) or with semisolid bulk, the gastrocolic reflex triggers the impulse to pass stool. Gas will also trigger it, which accounts at times for passing huge amounts of wind (flatus) without stool. (A large volume of gas in the gut can lead to cramps, since it is relatively compressed, hence expands the gut to discomfort.)

For that reason, the administration of bulk-forming laxatives, which are composed of certain gums, supply mass and start a peristaltic wave. They have a slippery feel, though not oily, and when in contact with water they expand, give bulk, and dissolve partially to make a thick solution. Being indigestible they are not absorbed. Bulk-forming laxatives remain in the gut until, when mixed with the intestinal contents, they are expelled together with the fecal matter in passing stool. Bulk laxatives, as psyllium seed derivatives, are taken with water. (Emulsions with mineral oil, as emulsions of mineral oil with psyllium, or chondrus [Irish moss] are also available, but those emulsions contain little bulk-producing laxatives and large proportions of mineral oil. They have fewer disadvantages than mineral oil.) Bulk-forming laxatives are not stimulant laxatives. Their sheer bulk stimulates the gastrocolic or the gastroileal reflex to facilitate passing stool.

Another advantage inherent in the use of bulk-forming laxatives resides in cases where it is undesirable to stimulate the gut.

Bulk-forming laxative preparations are particularly suitable for older people, provided that they do not need an intestinal stimulant stronger than that given by bulk. Some preparations contain equal quantities of psyllium derivative and dextrose; the latter has a caloric value and therefore should be used cautiously in a diabetic diet. Another variant is in an effervescent form—and you pay for the pleasure of effervescence by taking about 250 mg. sodium per dose. The effectiveness is the same; it may be merely more pleasant to take, though the noneffervescent psyllium hydrocolloid is not unpleasant.

Methylcellulose is a cellulose product used for bulk production as a laxative. It is available in the form of tablets which are taken with water. Sodium carboxymethylcellulose is quite similar. These celluloses are not found as mineral oil emulsions; also, they do not produce the type of bulk that other bulk-forming laxatives (psyllium derivatives) do.

If bulk-forming products are adequate, they are generally preferable to mineral oil emulsions, or laxatives. In fact, bulk-forming laxatives are not laxatives at all, but facilitate bowel movements by the slippery bulk they produce in the intestine and colon when taken with water.

SALINE LAXATIVES

These substances are salts that are freely soluble in water, which produces their laxative effect. They differ from bulk-producing laxatives in that they fill the gut with water by preventing the absorption of water by the intestine. This also triggers a reflex, urging expulsion. The saline laxatives act quickly, usually in 3 to 5 hours, depending on their dose.

The saline laxatives are (a) magnesium sulfate, better known as epsom salt; (b) sodium sulfate or Glauber's salt; (c) sodium phosphate, or effervescent sodium phosphate; (d) citrate of magnesium solution; and (e) disposable enemas which are sodium phosphate solutions given rectally.

These salts are always taken dissolved in water. Some are effervescent; others are not. They should be taken with one or two full glasses of water to increase palatability, to provide water for expulsion, and to prevent relative dehydration, for otherwise they draw much water from the tissues.

Saline laxatives have an advantage in that their effect is comparatively rapid, and expulsion of intestinal contents is as complete as, or more copious than, that obtained with stimulating laxatives. Much of the volume, of course, is due to water. Perhaps they offer a psychological satisfaction in that the "cleaning-out" process shows a greater volume of watery stool. However, due to their rapidity of action they have an advantage in cases of food poisoning, when laxation is required.

Milk of magnesia acts more slowly and less vigorously. It is favored as a mild laxative.

While glycerine suppositories (rectal) are not saline laxatives, they work in much the same way, as they draw water from the tissues (glycerine is hygroscopic). The volume and irritation cause the urge to move bowels. While saline laxatives start working in the small intestine, glycerine suppositories work much lower—at the sigmoid and the near end of the colon.

Laxatives are at times taken to "clean out" because such

"cleaning-out" action is believed to be desirable when there is abdominal pain. *That is just the time they should not be taken,* unless a physician has prescribed a laxative. The reason is that abdominal pain, nausea, or vomiting may be due to an inflammation of the appendix. The more-or-less vigorous peristalsis that most laxatives produce (particularly stimulating laxatives) may rupture the appendix, resulting in peritonitis.

While ordinarily there is little or no danger in taking a laxative occasionally, it must not be forgotten that taking them with greater frequency precludes the setting up and observing of a pattern. Moving bowels is greatly dependent upon establishing a regular time, whether at the moment an urge does or does not exist.

Taking a laxative instead of attending to a dietary improvement which includes roughage (vegetables)—assuming that roughage is not contraindicated—is also militating against the establishment of a dietary pattern.

There are other reasons why laxatives, generally, may have untoward effects. One is that producing watery stools may draw along needed electrolytes—sodium, potassium, and other ions or minerals which are needed in metabolism. Or they may dehydrate; this particularly applies to stimulant or saline laxatives taken frequently.

Pure mineral oil or laxatives containing mineral oil may interfere with the absorption of certain nutritional elements, as fat-soluble vitamins. Also, droplets of mineral oil left in the throat may be inhaled and can set up an irritation in the lungs. It should not be given to people who are recovering from stroke, as their swallowing function may be impaired. Combinations of agar and mineral oil, psyllium seed and mineral oil, or chondrus (Irish moss) and mineral oil are preferable for that reason, since these drawbacks are reduced with these preparations, as compared with pure mineral oil.

There is no particular drawback to the stool softeners, such as preparations consisting of dioctyl sodium sulfosuccinate, except those cautions against the use of laxatives generally, as a habit. In fact, if there is sufficient muscle tone and peristaltic action which propels the intestinal contents downward, stool softeners are preferable to those containing a stimulant laxative combined with the stool softener for older people; many of them need laxation, due to inactivity and other reasons having to do with their life-style.

The drawback to bulk-forming laxatives, which are otherwise at times preferable, is twofold: (1) if the bulk-producing product is a mineral oil emulsion it has the detriment associated with mineral oil, though not in the same measure as plain mineral oil; (2) if taken as a dry gum or psyllium seed, it may produce obstruction and impaction, especially if not taken with sufficient water. A small amount of water may be enough to wet the gum to bring out its adhesive quality to produce a solid plug or lump—hence obstruction in the gullet, or stomach. If there is a history of intestinal obstruction, they should not be used.

With cathartics containing sodium salts there may occur another disadvantage. If more or less concentrated solutions are taken, they remain in the stomach until enough water has been absorbed from the body to cause their downward trek. Therefore they should be taken with ample water. But there is some absorption of the saline laxative by the body. What the body does absorb from saline laxatives are the ions—sodium, potassium, magnesium. Ordinarily, such absorption is not a problem; in fact tablets containing salt (sodium chloride) are taken during periods of intense heat and perspiration to supply the salt lost during perspiration.

However, in people with edema and those with high blood pressure the intake of salt is restricted (to reduce the amount of sodium in the body). Sodium increases water retention. Thus when sodium is absorbed from a saline laxative, the purpose is defeated. Hence, if you must restrict your sodium intake, and you insist on having a saline laxative for some reason or other, do not take one containing sodium (see labels), but instead take magnesium sulfate, also known as epsom salts.

Here you may well be on the horns of a dilemma, though one that is not overcommon. Why? Because if you have an inadequate kidney function, the magnesium ion—part of magnesium sulfate—is not excreted as rapidly as it should be. Hence it accumulates and raises the blood level of magnesium. If that becomes high enough the result may be depression of respiration or of blood pressure to an unacceptable low. Ordinarily, the average amount of magnesium is relatively nontoxic. Magnesium is also an ingredient in milk of magnesia, citrate of magnesium solution (which also contains sodium), certain antacids containing magnesium trisilicate or magnesium carbonate or oxide, but in those preparations the magnesium is less available.

MYTHS

Myths pertaining to the passing of stool are numerous—and many are scatological. Some myths, however, are close to truths, or partial truths. For example, one belief is that if a bowel movement induced by a laxative was copious, it was high time for it. Since succeeding bowel movements will be sparse, a laxative will be necessary again quite soon. The facts are these: (a) A copious movement means that much water was extracted from the tissues, which added to the volume of the stool. It does not mean that it was "high time for a physic." (b) Several succeeding bowel movements will be relatively sparse, normally so, because they will not have the addition of water nor the stimulus of laxatives. (c) A laxative is not necessary when stools are sparse. That depends on many factors, among which are the type of diet, the amount of liquid consumed, the nervous function. It is of interest to note that in many African tribes, the amount of stool passed is bulky, large, porous and frequent—usually two or three times daily—but not watery. The reason is their diet, which is high in vegetable matter, low in proteins, and particularly low in carbohydrates.

Another myth states that when an individual is excited he is not constipated. Though by and large this is true, excitement is not recommended as a remedy for constipation (nor is depression recommended to cure diarrhea).

A third myth deals with purification. Indeed, stool does not serve a purpose in the body and should be discharged. Unduly long storage of stool in the rectum does tend to affect comfort, reduce appetite, etc. However, the feeling of relief after a copious or long-held movement is illusory—it is not a health sign but merely a return to what should be a normal feeling of well-being. This is reminiscent of Dryden's comments that the greatest happiness of man is absence of pain. But this notion has the psychological overtones of purification rites, which have their roots deep in the atavistic memories of man.

A health cult has grown up about stool. Many esoteric foods are sold for inducing it. If these foods supply predominantly roughage, which is what they do, their advantage over vegetables escapes us. When a food—health food or other food—grows into the size of a cult, it is time to reevaluate it. And reevaluation will usually find it wanting.

However, certain foods, such as bran or vegetables, which are indeed adequate as a part of the normal diet, may be contraindicated in certain conditions, and your physician should be consulted in those cases.

If Your Need Is for a Laxative Against Constipation:

Look for Products Containing the Following Ingredients:

- Milk of magnesia
- Bulk-forming laxatives
- Dioctyl sodium sulfosuccinate
- Salines, as
  - citrate of magnesium solution
  - disposable enema of sodium phosphate
- Stimulants, as
  - phenolphthalein
  - cascara
  - danthron
  - senna derivative

Avoid the Following Ingredients:

- Plain mineral oil (preferably avoided)
- Psyllium products (unless taken with at least a glassful of water)
- Saline laxatives containing sodium if you must restrict the intake of sodium

NAMES OF PRODUCTS

STIMULANT LAXATIVES

Agoral (Warner-Chilcott)—Contains phenolphthalein and mineral oil in emulsion.

Alophen Pills (Parke, Davis)—Contains aloin 1/4 grain, belladonna 1/24 grain, powdered ipecac 1/15 grain, phenolphthalein 1/2 grain.

Black Draught Syrup (Chattem)—Contains senna and rhubarb.

Caroid and Bile Salts (Sterling)—Contains caroid 75 mg., capsicum 6.48 mg., dried whole bile 70 mg., phenolphthalein 32.4 mg., and extract cascara sagrada 48 mg.

Carter's Little Pills (Carter-Wallace)—Contains podophyllum and aloes.

Correctol Tablets (Pharmaco)—Contains dioctyl sodium sulfosuccinate 100 mg. and 1 gr. yellow phenolphthalein.

Dialose Plus (Stuart)—Contains oxyphenisatin acetate 3 mg., dioctyl sodium sulfosuccinate 100 mg., and sodium carboxymethylcellulose 400 mg.

Dr. Edward's Olive Tablets (Plough)—Contains podophyllin, aloin, and extract of cascara.

Dorbantyl Capsules (Riker)—Contains danthron 25 mg. and dioctyl sodium sulfosuccinate 50 mg.

Espotabs Tablets (Combe)—Contains yellow phenolphthalein.

Ex-Lax (Ex-Lax Co.)—Contains yellow phenolphthalein.

Feen-a-Mint Gum Tablets (Pharmaco)—Contains yellow phenolphthalein.

Gentlax Granules (Purdue Frederick)—Contains senna concentrate and guar gum.

Innerclean Granules (Innerclean Co.)—Contains senna, frangula, psyllium, and agar.

Kondremul with Phenolphthalein (Smith, Miller & Patch)—Contains phenolphthalein and Irish moss with mineral oil emulsion. (Also available plain, and with cascara.)

Nature's Remedy Tablets (Lewis-Howe)—Contains aloe and cascara.

Peri-Colace (Mead Johnson)—Contains casanthranol 30 mg. and dioctyl sodium sulfosuccinate 100 mg.

Petrogalar (Wyeth)—Contains phenolphthalein and mineral oil in emulsion. (Also available plain, with cascara, or with milk of magnesia.)

Regutol Tablets (Pharmaco) —Contains dioctyl sodium sulfosuccinate 100 mg. and calcium pantothenate 50 mg.

Senokap DSS Capsules (Purdue Frederick)—Contains senna and dioctyl sodium sulfosuccinate.

Senokot Granules (Purdue Frederick) —Contains senna.

Senokot Powder (Purdue Frederick)—Contains senna with psyllium.

Senokot Syrup (Purdue Frederick) —Contains extract of senna.

Zilatone Tablets (Breon)—Contains phenolphthalein, dried whole bile, extract cascara, pancreatin, pepsin, and capsicum.

LUBRICANT LAXATIVES

Colace Capsules (Mead Johnson)—Consists of dioctyl sodium sulfosuccinate (DOSS), in capsules of 50 mg. or 100 mg.

Dialose (Stuart) —Contains dioctyl sodium sulfosuccinate 100 mg. and sodium carboxymethylcellulose 400 mg.

Dioctyl Sodium Sulfosuccinate Capsules or Tablets (Various Manufacturers) —Consists of DOSS. (DOSS is commonly available in a combination with stimulant laxatives; hence these combinations are listed under Stimulant Laxatives.)

Mineral Oil Enema (Fleet)—A disposable, plastic enema device for single use, containing mineral oil, for rectal administration, to lubricate and soften hard stools in the rectum.

BULK-FORMING LAXATIVES

Effersyllium (Stuart)—Contains hydrophyllic mucilloid of psyllium, in an effervescent form. Note: contains sodium.

Konsyl (Burton, Parsons)—Consists of hydrophyllic mucilloid of psyllium.

L.A. Formula (Burton, Parsons)—Contains equal parts of Konsyl (see above) and dextrose. There is no advantage or disadvantage to this product as compared with Konsyl, except that it contains half the amount of bulk-producing material, and it suspends better in water.

Metamucil (Searle)—Consists of hydrophylic mucilloid of psyllium and dextrose, equal parts.

Metamucil Instant Mix (Searle)—Same as Metamucil, but in effervescent form—requires no mixing, not that mixing is a hard task. Note: contains 250 mg. sodium per dose.

Mucilose Flakes Concentrated (Winthrop)—Consists of cellulose from psyllium.

Mucilose Granules Special Formula (Winthrop)—Contains psyllium concentrate and dextrose, equal parts.

Sof-Cil (Zemmer)—Contains psyllium mucilloid with dioctyl sodium sulfosuccinate.

SALINE LAXATIVES

Citrate of Magnesia (Various Manufacturers)—Contains magnesium citrate in solution.

Fleet Brand Enema (Fleet)—A disposable, plastic enema device for single use, containing sodium acid phosphate and sodium phosphate, for the rapid emptying of stools from the rectum.

Haley's M-O (Sterling)—Contains milk of magnesia with 25% mineral oil.

Milk of Magnesia (Various Manufacturers)—Contains magnesium hydroxide in suspension.

Phospho-Soda (Fleet)—Contains sodium biphosphate and sodium phosphate in solution.

Sal Hepatica (Bristol-Myers)—Contains sodium bicarbonate, citric acid, and monosodium phosphate.

DIARRHEA AND ANTIDIARRHEALS

DEFINITION

Diarrhea is the discharge of watery stools, usually repeated several times an hour to several times a day. Thus, diarrhea is as much a matter of frequency as well as of liquidity. It is often, though not necessarily, accompanied by abdominal cramps.

CAUSE

Diarrhea is a complex phenomenon and may be due to one or a number of causes. Acute diarrhea has a sudden onset, with little or no previous history, and the expulsion of frequent watery stools and gas may or may not be associated with weakness or loss of appetite. Such an acute episode of diarrhea may be due to an emotional upset or to an infection, more frequently to a bacterial or viral intestinal infection such as a cold. Or it may stem from having eaten food that is toxic or develops a toxin ("spoiled food"), as in a *Salmonella* infection. Then too, diarrhea may occur because of a change in the nature of the bacterial population of the intestine after antibiotic treatment. It may also follow treatment by x-rays. Some believe that food allergy can produce diarrhea; others deny it.

DISCUSSION AND CAUTIONS

While constipation usually does not require the regular use of laxatives, diarrhea usually does require ongoing treatment to ameliorate it. Moreover, diarrhea, except when it occurs casually or infrequently, may and often does require professional help to determine why it occurred and the manner in which it should be treated. Constipation rarely kills; diarrhea, depending on its cause, more frequently does. In fact, diarrhea in infants or young children can be rapidly fatal if untreated.

An acute episode of anything is one that occurs suddenly and usually has strong and definite symptoms. Chronic diarrhea—one that has reasonably mild symptoms but is long lasting or sporadically recurs—paradoxically usually is more serious. (Of course, chronic diarrhea may have its acute episode or happening, which then improves and returns to its chronic state.)

Chronic constipation is responsive to a reeducation of bowel habits or, at worst, to laxatives. Except for impaction, it is not life-threatening. But chronic diarrhea may be a symptom of a life-threatening condition—as, for example, in ulcerative colitis, an inflammation of part of the small intestine (regional enteritis); infestation with parasites; diverticulitis; or in one of the varieties of cancer. Thus, an *on-again, off-again* (chronic) diarrhea should be diagnosed and treated by a physician. Even if it is bearable, it may lead to secondary problems. These may be malnutrition due to impairment of absorption of nutrients by the small intestine through the rapid transit of food through the alimentary tract; loss of weight, which may not be merely loss of water through watery stools but also loss of muscle mass due to malnutrition; anomalies of nerve function due to loss of valuable electrolytes, as sodium, potassium, magnesium, etc.; or dehydration due to excessive loss of water and salts, if they are not replaced.

No attempt should be made to treat chronic diarrhea with over-the-counter drugs or otherwise. This should be done by a physician.

In treating your own acute happening of diarrhea which does *not* have a history of regular occurrence, you have access to a number of effective remedies. But before you choose your remedy think back: did you have a particularly trying time with your boss, partner, or wife? There is no shame in having diarrhea in response to emotional upsets. The gastrointestinal tract is highly responsive to emotional stimuli, and it can reflect many different feelings. Diarrhea is an accentuation or exaggeration of the motor activity of the colon—just the opposite of constipation, which is a depression of that activity. Such an accentuation of colonic activity can occur with overstimulation, irritation, or excitement. If you can place the origin—whether excitement or food toxin or viral infection—you will be able to handle the problem more intelligently.

In fact, with repeated exposure to a chain of emotional upsets resulting in diarrhea, a more hazardous condition known as the irritable colon syndrome can develop. It is not unusual to find such events as a man consistently refusing to take a Sunday afternoon drive with his wife because he develops diarrhea. This is not his response to his wife's Sunday dinner but to her abrasive driving directions. There is no over-the-counter remedy for diarrhea precipitated by such happenings, which is really an accentuation or speeding up of normal function of the intestine and colon. What remedies can be used in such a case? A choice can be made: (a) ask your doctor for a sedative to be used after returning from the drive, or (b) stop driving with your wife.

INGREDIENTS

To alleviate acute diarrhea in adults, paregoric is an excellent remedy in teaspoonful doses to be taken after each bowel movement. In addition, other adsorbent or binding substances are available, such as aluminum hydroxide gel, and more particularly kaolin, an inactive clay, or pectin from fruit rinds. These substances adsorb irritants—bacteria and toxins that may have been taken in food—and they take them along in their alimentary trek to excretion. Toxins may also have been elaborated in the intestine by coli or putrefaction bacteria. Kaolin or pectin protects by forming a film on the intestinal walls. However, another inactive clay, attapulgite, is superior to kaolin in its adsorptive effect due to its greater surface area, hence adsorptive capacity. Unfortunately, only one product available over-the-counter without prescription contains it. The trouble with kaolin and pectin is that they adsorb also the salutory bacteria of the intestinal tract which are necessary for digestion as well as for the normal endogenous vitamin synthesis in the intestine. (To reestablish these bacteria, tablet preparations containing *Lactobacillus acidophilus* are available.)

Hyoscyamine, hyoscine, and atropine are all alkaloids of belladonna and supplement the adsorptive effect of kaolin, by reducing spasm of the intestine, which is the source of painful discomfort. These substances make an excellent addition to antidiarrheal products.

Preparations containing bismuth subcarbonate are also useful, but kaolin and pectin are preferable because they are highly adsorbent. In the event of food poisoning—though self-diagnosis is unreliable—powdered charcoal is excellent, due to its immense adsorbing facility.

These antidiarrheal drugs should be taken until the first sign of a formed stool is observed. Then they should be stopped immediately to avoid constipation. A low-residue diet (no vegetables) is recommended by some for several days after a bout of acute diarrhea to prevent further irritation, though others believe that such restriction is unnecessary. If diarrhea is due to allergy to some food, which some believe to be one cause, an attempt should be made to determine after what food diarrhea occurs and to eliminate it from the diet.

Diarrhea due to a viral infection is self-limited and is perhaps best treated with kaolin-pectin adsorbents.

Diarrhea after antibiotic treatment is best treated by your physician, by stopping the antibiotic.

MYTHS

Many myths have arisen as to the cause of diarrhea. As with other myths, some of them carry various degrees of truth or half-truth. For example, the traditional combinations of sour pickles and ice cream, or chocolate and fish, are often reputed to be sure to produce diarrhea. These are myths indeed. If for some reason you like the combination of sour pickles and ice cream, continue and choose your own ice cream flavors.

Another theory has it that cold drinks taken while overheated produce diarrhea. That is no myth but a fact—not because it "spoils the stomach," but because the sudden chill increases motor activity of the colon, like excitement.

A third notion concerns cabbage as causing diarrhea. It may. Cabbage, in common with other vegetable foods, particularly when raw and eaten in quantity, can well produce mild diarrhea because the large bulk produces a sense of fullness which triggers the ileogastric reflex to move bowels.

A fourth myth says that prunes produce diarrhea. They may, but usually only when taken in considerably large quantities—say, about a pound. The reason is that prunes contain acetphenolisatin, which is exactly one of the stimulating laxatives used in modern products.

If Your Need Is for a Product Against Diarrhea:

Look for Products Containing the Following Ingredients:

- Paregoric (not available without prescription in some states; see note on paregoric below)
- Attapulgite
- Kaolin
- Pectin
- Belladonna alkaloids
- Activated charcoal

NAMES OF PRODUCTS

Donnagel (Robins)—Each fluid ounce contains kaolin 6 gm., pectin 142 mg., hyoscyamine sulfate 0.1037 mg., atropine sulfate 0.0194 mg., hyoscine hydrobromide 0.0065 mg., sodium benzoate, and 3.8% alcohol.

Kao-Con—Kaopectate Concentrate (Upjohn)—Each fluid ounce contains kaolin 9 gm. and pectin 200 mg.

Kaopectate (Upjohn)—Each fluid oz. contains kaolin 6 gm. and pectin 130 mg.

Paregoric (Various Manufacturers)—Contains opium, camphor, and alcohol. Not available in some states without a prescription, and this is likely to be a national order in the near future.

Pargel (Parke, Davis)—Each fluid oz. contains kaolin 6 gm. and pectin 130 mg.

Quintess (Lilly)—Contains activated attapulgite 3 gm. and colloidal activated attapulgite 0.9 gm.

INDIGESTION AND DIGESTANTS

DEFINITION

We wish we could clearly define indigestion. The difficulty resides in the fact that what is *considered* indigestion may be one or more of a number of sensations relating to the stomach —indefinite mild discomfort, sense of fullness, belching, at times nausea, or a mild pain in the pit of the stomach. By and large, indigestion is commonly considered as almost any stomach discomfort, especially after eating. (See also *Stomach*

Upset and Antacids.) And it is commonly ascribed by the one who complains of it to incomplete digestion.

CAUSE

Indigestion may be due to incomplete digestion of food before the stomach is emptied, especially when it occurs in those of middle age or older. More frequently, however, it may be due to (a) overeating and distending the stomach, (b) swallowing air, which may be ballooning the stomach or the foodpipe, (c) irritation due to excessive secretion of stomach acid, (d) emotional upset, (e) intolerance to certain foods, which is unpredictable. Such intolerance is the phenomenon in which certain foods cause abdominal discomforts to certain people. These foods are not really in themselves indigestible.

There may be more serious causes, such as stomach ulcer or obstruction or thickening of the portion of the stomach that adjoins the intestine (pylorus), which is next to the duodenum. Or stomach pain may be a "referred" pain. Referred pain is a pain occurring in a different part of the body than the seat of the trouble, due to a common nerve pathway. Pain in the stomach may actually arise from malfunction of the heart, or liver, or even infections of the urinary tract, or chronic gallbladder disease.

DISCUSSION AND CAUTIONS

It is unreasonable to expect any one drug to be useful for "indigestion" when it can be due to so many possible causes. The reason for the discomfort, especially if it is frequent, should be sought and treated by a physician. He may find that the so-called gas and indigestion is due merely to swallowing air—a frequent event and not consciously done. Or he may need to distinguish it from chronic gallbladder disease or hiatal hernia, or even find that an antacid may well be indicated. How soon after eating the discomfort occurs, whether immediately or delayed, may be significant in the diagnosis.

Paradoxically, an appreciable number of people have such discomfort not because of excess stomach acid but because of a paucity of it—they simply do not have enough. This occurs more often in older people. In that case the administration of dilute hydrochloric acid, which is further diluted with water, may dispose of the "acid stomach" belching and discomfort after eating.

But an unusually large number of stomach discomforts are due to psychosomatic causes. In describing the symptoms, it becomes a psycho*semantic* problem. Whether psychosomatic or psychosemantic, the common phrase "it turns my stomach" becomes almost literal, when, beset with interpersonal problems, a person begins his meal boiling with rage or frustration. In fact, many products for indigestion, available on prescription only, contain belladonna to reduce spasm or a sedative to reduce tension. The objective is to ameliorate the emotional component of indigestion or digestive discomfort.

INGREDIENTS

In the attempt to ameliorate indigestion, a number of products are offered. Certain antacids, particularly the effervescent ones, are often used with success in casual and mild discomforts. More particularly, there is a class of products called digestants, containing digestive enzymes, purported to help digestion of proteins, carbohydrates, or fats. Many such digestants, containing varying proportions and kinds of digestive enzymes, are available over-the-counter without a prescription.

The aim of using the digestive enzymes is to supplement a diminished secretion of digestive enzymes which are normally adequately elaborated in the gastrointestinal tract. But there is a clear difference of opinion as to the value of such enzyme preparations. Some believe they are without merit.

If you have digestive discomfort, bear in mind that there are various conditions to which it may be due. A recurring condition or a continuing one does need the opinion of a physician to diagnose, prevent or ameliorate. However, for the occasional occurrence, an antacid may be ameliorative (see *Stomach Upset and Antacids*).

Because indigestion may have any number of causes, there can be no one dietary recommendation. Generally, eat those foods that you are likely to tolerate.

If Your Need Is for a Product Against Indigestion:

(See *Stomach and Abdominal Discomfort*)

HELMINTHIASIS (WORMS) AND ANTHELMINTICS

DEFINITION

Helminthiasis is an infestation of the body by worms. Worms can infest almost any tissue—lungs, liver, even heart. Infestation, particularly in children, with pinworms, also known as seatworms or threadworms (enterobiasis or oxyuriasis), or with roundworms (ascariasis) is localized in the intestine, from which the worms migrate downward into the rectum and anus. An anthelmintic is an agent that is used in the treatment of worm infestation, either by killing them at some stage of their life, or by causing them to be expelled from the intestinal tract, or both.

CAUSE

Infestations.

Perhaps half of the population of the world plays host to worms, which produce a variety of diseases. Some of them are life-threatening. Infestation with pinworms and roundworms—to which we will limit this section because remedies for other worm diseases are not obtainable over-the-counter without prescription—is spread by ingestion of infected food or by poor hygiene habits. Eating candy does not cause worms.

DISCUSSION AND CAUTIONS

People should not be content that they have diagnosed worms because a child has itching of the anus and does not gain weight at the rate he should. Diagnosis of worm diseases is a combination of clinical signs, but without a laboratory diagnosis there cannot be certainty.

Therefore, a physician should be consulted if there is a suspicion that a child or other members of the family harbor worms. To eradicate the infestation and to prevent recurrence of pinworms, it is highly desirable to treat all members of the family living with the infested child. Fastidious hygienic practices should be observed, such as cleansing the anus with medicated disposable wipes after passing stool, sanitizing the toilet seat, the toilet bowl, and hands and nails. To prevent cross-infestation, paper towels should be used and burned after use. To prevent infecting other members of the family or reinfecting the child, anal hygiene must go to considerable lengths with respect to underwear (wear it under pajamas, wash separately and disinfect). Special care must also be taken in handling food and with use of flatware at the table.

INGREDIENTS

Among the many kinds of worm infestations are those with hookworm, whipworm and tapeworm, and grave conditions such as schistosomiasis or filariasis brought about by other parasites. All these surely require care by a physician, who can prescribe one or more of the many drugs that are available.

However, we are definitely considering anthelmintics as information, not recommendation. We are limiting our discussion to drugs available over-the-counter without prescription, for controlling only pinworms and roundworms. It is always a question of balancing the toxicity of an anthelmintic on the human body with its effectiveness against worms. Among anthelmintics for pinworms and roundworms, two substances stand out: gentian violet and hexylresorcinol.

Gentian violet is the oldest known and is a relatively nontoxic and reasonably efficient anthelmintic. It is effective against pinworms and is used daily for a two-week period.

Hexylresorcinol is effective against roundworms and pinworms, is reasonably nontoxic and efficient, and is also given for a two-week period. It is preferable because it is active against a greater variety of worms.

We are not supplying the customary listing of the few over-the-counter products available, because we clearly believe that if worms are suspected, a physician should both diagnose whether this is so and treat the worm infestation if present.

If Your Need Is for a Product Against Helminthiasis (Worms):

Do not take anything—see your doctor.

HEMORRHOIDS

DEFINITION

Hemorrhoids (piles) are veins in the rectum which have become and remain dilated or swollen and inflamed. Usually more than one vein is involved in the small space. They may be compared to varicose veins. Hemorrhoids can be internal (just inside the rectum) or external (when they slip beyond the anus and protrude).

CAUSE

Many causes are given for the development of hemorrhoids. Among the most frequent ones is habitual constipation, which makes straining at stool necessary. Even continued diarrhea, producing irritation, may be a cause. Coughing can worsen hemorrhoids. Prolonged standing or sitting, which affects the hydrostatic events in the veins in the rectum, and also poor circulation in the anal region are also given as causes. Lifting weights and intense coughing exaggerate the discomfort of hemorrhoids. Increased abdominal pressure, as during pregnancy, or bearing down during delivery may make hemorrhoids appear which were not troublesome before. And possibly there is a constitutional predisposition to hemorrhoids due to structural characteristics of the veins of the rectum. One possible cause, arising out of liver cirrhosis, is that there is scarring of the liver, which causes pressure on the large veins that pass through it, and these pressure changes can be reflected by back pressure to the rectal veins, causing hemorrhoids.

DISCUSSION AND CAUTIONS

The rectum is the lowest extremity of the alimentary (digestive) tract. Hence disturbances relating to any part of the tract can well affect hemorrhoids. For example, some foods that have passed the alimentary tract often affect hemorrhoids: the skin of hot red peppers is undigested, usually indigestible, and is excreted as such. The result may be that there is a burning sensation in the rectum.

The hardness of stools passed affects hemorrhoids, too. There is considerable irritation to hemorrhoids when straining to pass hard stool, from two standpoints: (1) the irritation of a hard object rubbed against them, and (2) the back pressure of blood created by straining, which further enlarges them.

But hemorrhoids have a social complexion, for in our culture they are associated with a scatological subject. While buttocks do not share in that social opprobrium—note sculptures and paintings of nudes—there is no work of art in which the anus is pictured.

Because it is not normally socially acceptable to mention the rectum or anus—there may be penis envy but no anus envy—disorders of the rectum and anus are not usually discussed. Hence, they tend to be neglected, and the lay person is even less informed about that part of the body and its function than about sex. (About sex he has at least misinformation *—and truth springs more readily from error than from secrecy or confusion.*)

If constipation occurs due to a change of diet ordered for a reason other than hemorrhoids, mineral oil-containing laxatives, i.e., mineral oil emulsions with chondrus or agar, are preferable because they lend lubricity to the stool being expelled. Constipation increases discomfort of hemorrhoids.

However, before going farther we should raise some questions. Is it a hemorrhoid, a polyp, a fissure, or is the so-called hemorrhoid a clot in the rectal vein? These have to be differentiated, and only a physician can do so. It is good to have medical attention even if only to determine whether the problem actually is a hemorrhoid. If it is a clot—i.e., a thrombosed pile or hemorrhoid—it can be easily opened and the clot evacuated, which is often an office procedure.

There is a similar condition, wartlike growths called *condylomata acuminata* (singular, *condyloma*), that, while usually benign, can be distressing. They are ordinarily treated by a physician, requiring half a dozen or more applications. The big reason why a hemorrhoid should be diagnosed by a physician is to find whether it is a hemorrhoid or possibly cancer. In fact, hemorrhoids can sometimes result from an obstruction in the bowel higher up, causing distention of the hemorrhoidal veins. For that reason, anyone who develops hemorrhoids after the age of 40 should have a sigmoidoscopy and a barium enema for proper diagnosis.

Bright red blood streaking of the stool usually means that the hemorrhoid is external or internal and close to the anus. There is relief when the swelling goes down. Bleeding that is darker may be farther up.

Hemorrhoids are often associated with itching—*pruritus ani.* The itching is not a problem per se; it is the scratching that may infect ordinarily quiescent hemorrhoids.

A sufferer from hemorrhoids can do much to mitigate his discomforts. For example, if constipated, steps should be taken to make bowel movements soft, so that there is no straining at stool or trauma in passing stool. Roughage should be reduced—though not eliminated. Spices should be curtailed. Ordinarily, herbal spices, as dill, oregano, cinnamon, sage, thyme, parsley, even onions and a moderate amount of pepper, are not troublesome. But caraway, chili, curry, and crushed red pepper can raise havoc by anal burning.

Anal hygiene is a *sine qua non.* Warm applications after bowel movement can be easily used even when away from home, by wiping with a wad of toilet tissue saturated with warm water. At home, warm sitzbaths are helpful.

And such simple steps as increasing activity if one is sedentary, or sitting down when coughing, can reduce the acute pain and the feeling of generalized discomfort.

INGREDIENTS

Among the helpful remedies available over-the-counter without prescription to reduce discomfort from hemorrhoids are ointments and suppositories.

An ointment has the advantage of being applied by the index finger (never use a pile pipe!), which both brings the ointment to the painful site and, by the pressure of the finger, pushes the hemorrhoid back, though usually only partially.

The advantage of a suppository lies in the fact that, though when first inserted it slips up into the rectum, upon melting the ingredients seep down by gravity and friction to supply a more-or-less continuous supply of medication.

Aerosol sprays are convenient, but their disadvantage is that they touch only the external part of the rectum, and so may give only partial relief. We are not aware of advantages that rectal aerosol sprays may have.

A simple hemorrhoid remedy, though it does not have the advantages of medication that hemorrhoid ointments and suppositories have, is white petrolatum or Vaseline. When applied into the rectum by the finger, it lubricates and relieves hemorrhoidal pain engendered by friction when walking.

A number of ingredients used in hemorrhoid preparations are useful for relief, but they are not a cure.

Among the most important are those that contract small

blood vessels—vasoconstrictors. Ephedrine or ephedrine hydrochloride and phenylephrine hydrochloride are vasoconstrictors that are commonly used. It is good judgment to choose hemorrhoid ointments or suppositories that contain a vasoconstrictor.

Astringents are another group of substances that are constrictors, but they constrict tissue rather than blood vessels; they are not as efficient as *vaso*constrictors. Among astringents are tannic acid, bismuth subgallate, alum, zinc sulfate or zinc chloride, and, in a lesser measure, zinc oxide, which is a mild astringent but is essentially protective. Other bismuth salts (subcarbonate or subnitrate) are also protective as well as weakly astringent.

Another highly useful ingredient is a local anesthetic. It reduces both the pain sensation and the itching. The local anesthetics used include one of the following: pramoxine hydrochloride (Tronothane), diperodon hydrochloride (Diothane), benzocaine, tetracaine hydrochloride (Pontocaine), or dibucaine hydrochloride (Nupercaine). Benzyl alcohol is a much milder anesthetic. It is desirable to choose a hemorrhoidal ointment or suppository containing a local anesthetic. Belladonna is often an ingredient in ointments or suppositories. While it does not have a local anesthetic effect, it is a good additive because its antispasmodic effect does help to relieve pain.

Infections must be avoided. Avoid infection by practicing good anal hygiene. For that reason, when using an ointment or suppository, choose one that contains a bactericide or germicide. Here two different problems present themselves: (a) some of these products (as well as local anesthetics) are sensitizing, but that can usually be determined only upon trial and error; and (b) while some germicides "kill germs on contact," they do so very poorly in a fat vehicle—which is the vehicle used in hemorrhoidal ointments and suppositories. Nonetheless, it is wise to use a preparation that contains a germicide.

Among germicides are benzalkonium chloride, phenol, 8-

hydroxyquinoline, resorcin, and phenylmercuric nitrate or acetate (an excellent one).

Antiseptics or germicides of lesser effect are balsam Peru, boric acid, menthol; dependence should not be placed on them.

Another group of ingredients are surface-active agents (detergents), some of which are germicidal, but all of which lower surface tension, which may help the spread of ingredients into more intimate contact with the hemorrhoid. Tyloxapal (Triton A-20) and sodium lauryl sulfate are useful ones for that purpose, followed by benzalkonium chloride; the latter is also germicidal.

Some preparations claim to aid healing of the hemorrhoid. One, for example, contains cod liver oil, another vitamins A and D, a third a material called live yeast cell factor. While cod liver oil is an excellent healing agent on skin, the situation in hemorrhoids—where dilation and often breaks of a vein are involved—is a different matter. Cod liver oil does not heal hemorrhoids. On the "live yeast cell factor" there are distinct differences of opinion. Shark liver oil is similar to cod liver oil, and does not have specific hemorrhoid-curing quality, as far as is known.

Hemorrhoidal ointments and suppositories are an aid, often a comfort, and are clearly useful, provided that dietary and hygienic measures are used in addition and that constipation is avoided.

MYTH

A hot, wet teabag, exhausted from making tea, is an excellent application to sore hemorrhoids. *Fact:* yes and no. It is a good measure when other methods of relief are unobtainable. But do not use an "exhausted" teabag: part of the advantage lies in the astringent effect of the tannic acid of the tea. The moist heat is also comforting. Dip the teabag into hot water for a moment (to wet and heat thoroughly) and apply, if no other measure for relief is available.

If Your Need Is for a Product Against Hemorrhoids (Piles):

Look for Ointments or Suppositories Containing the Following Ingredients:

- Phenylephrine
- Ephedrine
- Bismuth subgallate
- Tannin
- Alum
- Benzocaine
- Dibucaine
- Belladonna
- Benzalkonium chloride
- Benzethonium chloride
- Phenylmercuric nitrate or acetate

Avoid the Following Ingredients:

- Aerosol form (unless hemorrhoid is external)

NAMES OF PRODUCTS

Note: Several products for hemorrhoids are available in two forms, both suppositories and ointments. While they carry the same name (as, for example, Nupercainal Ointment and Suppositories or Wyanoid Ointment and Suppositories) the formula of each form may not be the same. That is neither an advantage nor a detriment. But we make that point here to alert you to the situation. Thus, if a suppository is useful, an ointment may or may not have the same beneficial effect. Or, in fact, it may prove better. The only answer is trial—and perhaps error.

A & D Hemorrhoidal Suppositories (White Labs.)—Contains vitamins A and D, balsam Peru, bismuth subgallate, and zinc oxide.

Anusol Hemorrhoidal Suppositories (Warner-Chilcott)—Contains bismuth subgallate, bismuth resorcinol compound, benzyl benzoate, balsam Peru, zinc oxide, and boric acid.

Anusol Ointment (Warner-Chilcott)—Contains approximately the same formula as suppositories.

Calmol 4 Hemorrhoidal Suppositories (Leeming/Pfizer)—Contains cod liver oil, zinc oxide, bismuth subgallate, and balsam Peru.

Desitin Rectal Ointment (Leeming/Pfizer)—Contains zinc oxide, cod liver oil, and sodium lauryl sulfate.

Diothane Ointment (Richardson-Merrell)—Contains diperodon 1% and oxyquinoline benzoate 0.1%.

Humphreys Hemorrhoid Ointment (Humphrey Pharmacal)—Contains camphor, pyroligneous acid, benzocaine, witch hazel, and oil of rosemary.

Medicone Derma Ointment (Medicone Co.)—Contains benzocaine, oxyquinoline sulfate, menthol, zinc oxide, and ichthammol. (Same formula as Medicone Rectal Unguent but the latter contains balsam Peru instead of ichthammol, both about equal in mild antiseptic effect.)

Medicone Rectal Suppositories (Medicone Co.)—Contains benzocaine, oxyquinoline sulfate, zinc oxide, menthol, and balsam Peru.

Medicone Rectal Unguent (Medicone Co.)—Contains benzocaine, oxyquinoline sulfate, menthol, zinc oxide, and balsam Peru. (Same formula as Medicone Derma Ointment, but the latter contains ichthammol instead of balsam Peru; both are about equal in mild antiseptic effect.)

Medicone Rectal Wipes (Medicone Co.)—Contains benzalkonium chloride 0.02%, methyl paraben 0.15%, witch hazel 50%, and glycerine 10%.

Nemiroff Rectal Ointment (Nemiroff)—Contains zinc oxide, diperodon hydrochloride, bismuth subcarbonate, pyrilamine maleate, phenylephrine hydrochloride, in cod liver oil-petrolatum base.

Nupercainal Hemorrhoidal Suppositories (Madison/Ciba)—Contains nupercaine, zinc oxide, and bismuth subgallate.

Nupercainal Ointment (Madison/Ciba)—Contains 1% nupercaine (dibucaine hydrochloride).

Nupercainal Pain-Relief Cream (Madison/Ciba)—Same as above but 0.5% nupercaine (half strength).

Pazo Hemorrhoidal Ointment (Bristol-Myers)—Contains benzocaine, ephedrine sulfate, zinc oxide, camphor, and oil of eucalyptus.

Pazo Hemorrhoidal Suppositories (Bristol-Myers)—Contains same as ointment, above.

Perifoam Aerosol Spray (Holland Rantos)—Contains pramoxine hydrochloride and allantoin.

PNS Hemorrhoidal Suppositories (Sterling Drug)—Contains Pontocaine, Tetracaine, Neo-Synephrine (phenylephrine hydrochloride), tyloxapol, and bismuth subcarbonate.

Preparation H Hemorrhoidal Ointment (Whitehall)—Contains same as suppositories, below.

Preparation H Hemorrhoidal Suppositories (Whitehall)—Contains live yeast cell derivative—2,000 units skin respiratory factor (per ounce of suppository base), shark liver oil, and phenylmercuric nitrate 1:10,000.

Rectalgan Liquid (Ayerst)—Contains benzocaine, phenol, menthol, benzethonium chloride, 8-hydroxyquinoline, and methylparaben.

Tucks Ointment (Fuller)—Contains vitamins A and D and witch hazel.

Unguentine Hemorrhoidal Suppositories (Norwich)—Contains phenylmercuric acetate 0.012%, diperodon hydrochloride, aluminum hydrate, zinc carbonate, zinc acetate, zinc oxide, and boric acid.

Wyanoid Hemorrhoidal Ointment (Wyeth)—Contains zinc oxide, boric acid, ephedrine sulfate, benzocaine, and balsam Peru.

Wyanoids Hemorrhoidal Suppositories (Wyeth)—Contains zinc oxide, boric acid, ephedrine sulfate, extract belladonna, bismuth oxyiodide, bismuth subcarbonate, and balsam Peru.

PAIN

HEADACHE

DEFINITION

A headache is a pain in any part of the head. This obvious definition is modified by the fact that a feeling in the head of pressure or tightness, or other discomforts short of actual pain, are also loosely referred to as headache.

CAUSE

Is a headache a pain in the *head* or a pain in the mind? This is not meant to imply that a headache is imagined—we concede it is there. However, one of the most frequent causes of headache is emotional tension. The stress, fear, and apprehension associated with daily interplay among persons and happenings, and the resultant physical, emotional, and spiritual depletion or fatigue, come into play. One of the expressions of such interplay is headache.

Among the variety of serious causes of headache, which should not be self-treated, may be high blood pressure, poisoning, stroke, eye problems including glaucoma, allergy, alcoholism, tumor, migraine, anemia, pneumonia, influenza, measles, typhus or other serious infections, or neurological disturbances.

Other causes of headache, which can be self-treated, are colds and fever, eyestrain from concentration on painstaking work, dental problems that are being corrected, headache from a temporary flare-up of sinus inflammation, menstruation or premenstrual tension, tension of the muscles in back of the neck which often produces headache, or the headache that occurs when one is trying to stop smoking or drinking coffee.

Above all, headache often sets in when an individual's coping apparatus just gives out, and he therefore retreats into, takes refuge in, or is assailed by headache.

An acute headache in a person who rarely has them may mean that his response to his environment has slipped some cogs in his customary adjustment. Or it may mean that he is overwhelmed by an acute infection.

A person who has chronic headaches usually handles them reasonably adequately. But that is part of the problem. He should find out *why* he has chronic headaches. Some indications as to cause reside in the *frequency* with which they recur, and what events are associated with their recurrence. For example, getting a headache usually on Monday may well be due to drinking too much on weekends. It may be resentment at the prospect of spending the coming week at the scene of an eternal defeat—your work.

DISCUSSION AND CAUTIONS

No age or sex is spared the experience of headache. But more women complain of it than men, and suffer with it more frequently. This suggests that emotional volatility may be related to it.

And headaches differ: they may be diffused over the whole head, or they may be localized. The pain may be dull and achy or sharp and piercing. It may throb, or merely be a belt or zone of pain. None of these sites or kinds clearly suggest the reason for the headache, but in addition to a study of other events, they may point to a cause.

Sinus headache may be worse in the morning. A headache that appears toward the end of the day may more likely be a response to the troublesome events of the day, or it may be a result of eyestrain. Obviously, if self-treated without satisfaction or if it recurs frequently, professional attention should be sought. But above all, if light aggravates headache, if vision is impaired—i.e., if one sees double or has blind zones—or if headache is associated with vomiting, by all means get professional attention.

The situational, psychological, and cultural environment to which one responds with headache is suggested by the common phrases "I-get-a-headache-listening-to-him" or "You-give-me-a-pain-in-the-neck"; the muscle tension at the back of the neck often manifests itself as a headache.

INGREDIENTS

Relatively few substances are offered for headache. But they make up the ingredients in a vast number of products, available over-the-counter without prescription. These substances are predominantly aspirin, acetphenetidin (phenacetin), salicylamide, acetaminophen, and often caffeine. While each, except caffeine, shares a basic analgesic property, they differ in some respects which may make one preferable in certain instances, for certain people, and at certain times.

The above substances are usually combined—two or more, or all of them. In their behalf the claim is often made that these combinations give quicker or better pain relief than any one of them alone. There is considerable doubt that this is so. The reason for the doubt resides in the fact that these products are the sum of the ingredients—the effect being due to the sum of the quantities of the ingredients. For example, a mixture of 200 mg. each of aspirin, salicylamide, and acetaminophen will *probably* be no better than 600 mg. of any one of these ingredients.

Nonetheless, there is merit in these mixtures. One is based on the relative unpredictability of effect of any one of these ingredients in a given person: in some, aspirin may be the most preferable; in others, it may be acetaminophen that will be more effective. A mixture enables an individual to take an ingredient that he finds more effective. Otherwise, he will be obliged to experiment over a reasonable period of time, during which he takes comparable doses of each of these ingredients separately. And that, too, may have its merits.

Moreover, the statement that X is "slightly better" than Y has little or no merit. In such a subjective condition as headache there is no means of measuring slight variations. And there are too many other variables—such as time of day, severity of headache, ambient conditions, etc.—for slight variations to have any meaning.

In commenting upon the differences and safety factors among aspirin, acetaminophen, and salicylamide, we are referring to customary doses used over a limited period of time. In large doses and chronic use the above differ in their toxicities. Also, no categorical statements made in connection with these analgesics can apply, for many events take place in the metabolic conversions that often differ among people. (See also discussion on analgesics and table of differences among them, under *The Common Cold.*)

Aspirin is the analgesic most frequently used. It also has antipyretic as well as antiinflammatory effect, which means that it reduces fever and inflammation. Fever reduction may be useful when aspirin is used to mitigate the symptoms of colds, and reduction of inflammation when used in pain of arthritis. In headache, only the analgesic quality is the utilizable one. While aspirin is one of the safest of drugs when properly used, it has certain drawbacks. For example, some allergic people have a sensitivity to aspirin, and it can bring on an asthmatic attack; those people should never use it. (In fact, when buying an analgesic or a cold remedy, people sensitive to aspirin should carefully read the label to be assured that the product they plan to buy does not contain aspirin.)

Similarly, people who are taking anticoagulants—usually administered in the treatment of a heart attack or to reduce the clotting of blood in the veins of the leg (thrombophlebitis)—should not take aspirin. The reason is based on two phenomena: (a) aspirin also has a mild anticlotting effect, and the total effect of aspirin and anticoagulant can depress the clotting of the blood to the point that it may possibly result in hemorrhage; and (b) aspirin can interfere with a laboratory test (prothrombin time) which is used to monitor the effect of the anticoagulant and to guide continuing therapy with it.

Aspirin can irritate the stomach, especially in large doses. It may produce small points of bleeding in the stomach. Therefore it should not be used by people with stomach ulcer or those who are prone to irritation of the stomach (gastritis). If used, it can be taken in the form of buffered aspirin, which is a mixture of aspirin with an insoluble salt such as aluminum hydroxide or magnesium carbonate or hydroxide which mitigates its irritating effect on the stomach wall.

The claim is often made that aspirin works more rapidly if taken in the form of a liquid made by adding an effervescent tablet or salt in water. That is true—in solution it is absorbed more rapidly but its effect also dissipates more rapidly.

And another fact must be considered: among the ingredients that make an effervescent salt are sodium bicarbonate. Frequent use of bicarbonate increases the likelihood of alkalosis, makes the urine alkaline, hence can precipitate certain salts that are held in solution in the normally acid urine. The sodium of the sodium bicarbonate may put a load on the circulation of people with heart disease or high blood pressure. If taken in large quantities it may increase edema. This does not mean that the effervescent products should be avoided. But if used, the above factors should be kept in mind and weighed, particularly if used by people with heart disease or high blood pressure.

There are aspirin tablets on the market called timed-release tablets, or by similar names, which contain 10 or 20 grains of aspirin per tablet instead of the traditional 5 grains per tablet. The advantage claimed for them is that one dose lasts the whole day, paying out a gradual release of aspirin.

We fail to see the advantage that such delayed-effect tablets confer, except for the convenience of taking a dose once a day instead of two or three times a day. There is a counterbalancing advantage in taking regular 5-grain tablets, which release the aspirin and build a high blood and tissue level early, since it may stop the headache at once. If necessary to repeat the dose, it is not a high price to pay for the small inconvenience. But taken at bedtime, the delayed-effect tablets may have an advantage because their effect is of longer duration as compared with the regular 5-grain aspirin tablet. (See aspirin also under *Arthritis and Rheumatism* and *The Common Cold.*)

Salicylamide is a sort of first-cousin-once-removed to aspirin, but it is differently broken up in the body. Hence it may be used in conditions in which aspirin would not be the most suitable drug. (Aspirin—acetylsalicylic acid—is broken down in the body to salicylic acid, but salicylamide is not; it is excreted unchanged.) Salicylamide is about as readily absorbed as aspirin, and has about the same analgesic effect as aspirin, which makes its use in headache adequate. Salicylamide has a comparable fever-reducing (antipyretic) effect, which makes its use in colds and fever as satisfactory as that of aspirin, but that effect is not one sought in headache. Its antiinflammatory effect also favorably compares with aspirin, which makes it suitable in the treatment of symptoms of arthritis and rheumatism, but that effect is also not sought in headache. Salicylamide is more quickly absorbed than aspirin but its effect is not as long lasting.

Salicylamide does have certain advantages over aspirin: (a) it is not converted to a salicylate in the body, hence does not affect prothrombin time nor blood coagulability, and therefore can be used by people who are taking anticoagulants; (b) it does not cause stomach irritation and the stomach bleeding points that may ensue, hence may be used by people with stomach ulcer; (c) people who have an allergy to aspirin may use salicylamide and they do not react with asthma as they may to aspirin.

In most other respects, salicylamide resembles aspirin in its analgesic effect.

Acetphenetidin and Acetaminophen. A synonym for acetphenetidin is phenacetin. A synonym for acetaminophen is *N*-acetylpara-aminophenol or APAP.

Acetphenetidin and acetaminophen differ from aspirin and salicylamide. Both aspirin and salicylamide belong to the salicylate family, though like a black sheep salicylamide does not act the way a proper salicylate should. Both acetphenetidin and acetaminophen are members of an entirely different family—the para-aminophenols. The differences end in the way they are metabolized, and the similarities to aspirin and salicylamide begin when we consider the effect of both acetphenetidin and acetaminophen.

Acetphenetidin is by far the older member. Combined with aspirin and caffeine, it is an ingredient in the familiar APC (aspirin-phenacetin-caffeine) combination, under a variety of trademarked names. Both acetphenetidin and acetaminophen are antipyretic and analgesic but *not* antiinflammatory, which makes them unsuitable in arthritis but adequate for headache. Neither acetphenetidin nor acetaminophen is irritating, hence do not cause bleeding points in the stomach, but they are easily absorbed from the stomach. Either may be used by people sensitive to aspirin and neither affects blood coagulability.

But acetphenetidin may adversely affect hemoglobin, reducing its vital oxygen-carrying capacity, and cause methemoglobinemia. Acetphenetidin also carries a warning that it may cause kidney damage unless taken according to directions and should not be used for an excessive length of time.

We believe that it is as bad to alarm people without good reason as to mislead potential consumers with glowing but untruthful reports. For that reason we emphasize that while aspirin and acetphenetidin have their side effects, it does not mean that they are toxic or harmful when used knowledgeably and according to directions supplied on the label or accompanying package circular. It is generally safe to rely on the directions given in the package circulars. They are controlled by the Food and Drug Administration, and penalties may result for incompleteness or untruthful statements.

The dose of aspirin, salicylamide, acetphenetidin, or acetaminophen is about 5 grains (325 mg.), but acetphenetidin is usually taken in a dose half that amount. A single dose of a *combination* of the above is a total of about 5 grains (1 tablet). A preferable dose is a total of about 10 grains (2 tablets) containing two or more of the above ingredients.

Caffeine. Caffeine has long been an ingredient in APC combination tablets, accounting for the *C* in the name. Legend states that in the original APC combination, the *C* was for codeine. When the 1914 Harrison Narcotic Act came into effect, caffeine was substituted for the codeine. But the truth of that legend has not been ascertained. (APC tablets *with codeine* are available only on prescription.)

Caffeine is not an analgesic, yet has a good place in an analgesic combination. For example, coffee is often taken for a headache with apparently satisfactory results. This may be due to the hot drink itself or the relaxation during the short time that one sits having a cup of coffee or the change of attention from contemplation of the problems that may have brought on the headache. A cup of coffee contains 100 to 150 mg. caffeine.

Caffeine has definite pharmacological effects: (a) it stimulates the higher nervous centers (one reason for causing sleeplessness in some people); (b) it also stimulates motor muscles. Perhaps both effects render a lift to some people, and thus minister to a headache.

While a cup of coffee contains 100 to 150 mg. caffeine, the common APC tablet contains 15 to 30 mg. (¼ grain to ½ grain), too little to give a lift. Incidentally, some preparations contain caffeine citrate rather than caffeine. Caffeine citrate is a mixture of caffeine, which is an alkaloid, with citric acid to solubilize caffeine. But caffeine citrate is only half the strength of caffeine itself.

It is not possible to predict what the effect of caffeine will be in a given individual. Many people are sleepless, or have palpitations, after a cup of coffee. Others take a cup of coffee when they cannot sleep and fall asleep when they "hit the pillow."

Myth: A cola drink with aspirin "blows your mind." The fact: not true, but there is an effect to the combination. The stimulating effect of caffeine, which cola drinks contain, apparently is salubrious, while the aspirin exerts its regular analgesic effect. (Caffeine, in fact, has what may be considered a synergistic effect when used in combination with drugs for the treatment of migraine which are available on prescription only.)

Apparently nothing is absolutely safe, neither drugs nor foods. Various reports, some of which are definitely true, have appeared over the past several years that coffee (a) increases cholesterol, (b) precipitates heart attacks, (c) sensitizes the pancreas to put out more insulin, thus dropping blood sugar to uncomfortably low levels, and (d) increases stomach acidity, thus producing discomfort. While there is no doubt that these phenomena reported may well have been observed (interpretation is another matter), it seems that millions of cups of coffee are consumed daily, presumably, with less harm than the warnings would suggest. One drawback may have reduced the consumption of coffee—its considerable rise in price. To the health warnings we should add an economic one—it may produce slight malnutrition of the pocket. Stated differently, probably everything has its price which must be compared with the value expected to be received. One of the purposes of this book is to help the reader measure the price so that he can compare it with the value, i.e., the result he expects to achieve.

If Your Need Is for a Product Against Headache:

Look for Products Containing the Following Ingredients:

- Aspirin
- Phenacetin
- Salicylamide
- Acetaminophen

Avoid the Following Ingredients:

- Acetanilid

NAMES OF PRODUCTS

AGAINST HEADACHE

Alka-Seltzer Tablets (Miles)—Contains aspirin, monocalcium phosphate, sodium bicarbonate, citric acid; in solution it becomes sodium aspirin, calcium sodium phosphate, sodium bicarbonate, and sodium citrate.

Anacin Tablets (Whitehall)—Contains aspirin and caffeine.

Aspirin Tablets (Various Manufacturers)—Contains aspirin 5 grains.

Bayer Timed-Release Aspirin Tablets (Bayer)—Contains aspirin 10 grains.

B.C. Headache Powder (Block Drug)—Contains aspirin, salicylamide, and caffeine.

B.C. Tablets (Block Drug)—Contains aspirin, salicylamide, and caffeine.

Bromo Seltzer (Warner-Lambert)—Each capful contains acetaminophen 3 gr., phenacetin 2 gr., potassium bromide 2½ gr., caffeine, sodium bicarbonate, and citric acid.

Bufferin Tablets (Bristol-Myers)—Contains aspirin 5 gr. with aluminum-magnesium buffers.

Cope Tablets (Glenbrook)—Contains aspirin, methapyrilene fumarate, caffeine, aluminum-magnesium buffers. (Methapyrilene fumarate is an antihistamine, the side effect of which is drowsiness, hence relaxation.)

Coricidin Tablets (Schering)—Contains chlorpheniramine maleate 2 mg., aspirin 390 mg., and caffeine 30 mg. (Chlorpheniramine is an antihistamine.)

Empirin Compound Tablets (Burroughs Wellcome)—Contains phenacetin 2½ gr., aspirin 3½ gr., and caffeine ½ gr.

Excedrin Tablets (Bristol-Myers)—Contains acetaminophen 1½ gr., salicylamide 2 gr., aspirin 3 gr., and caffeine 1 gr.

Excedrin *PM* Tablets (Bristol-Myers)—Contains APAP 2½ gr., salicylamide, aspirin, methapyrilene fumarate. (Methapyrilene fumarate is an antihistamine, the side effect of which is drowsiness, hence relaxation.)

Fizrin Instant Alkalizer Seltzer (Glenbrook)—Contains aspirin 5 gr., sodium bicarbonate, sodium carbonate, citric acid; in solution it becomes sodium aspirin, sodium bicarbonate, sodium citrate.

Measurin Timed-Release Aspirin Tablets (Glenbrook)—Contains 10 gr. aspirin.

Nebs Tablets (Eaton)—Contains acetaminophen 325 mg. (5 gr.).

Tylenol Tablets (McNeil)—Contains acetaminophen 325 mg. (5 gr.).

Valadol Tablets (Squibb)—Contains acetaminophen 325 mg. (5 gr.).

Vanquish Caplets (Glenbrook)—Contains aspirin 227 mg., acetaminophen 194 mg., caffeine 33 mg., with aluminum-magnesium buffer.

ARTHRITIS AND RHEUMATISM

DEFINITIONS

Arthritis means inflammation of a joint. But what is commonly called arthritis and rheumatism is a group of several diseases or dysfunctions. Over-the-counter remedies available without prescription are for only two variants of these diseases. But we should make the distinction among the several kinds of arthritis and rheumatism, because one should know what type of arthritis or rheumatism he has, as treatments differ.

Rheumatoid arthritis may affect any joint. It is an inflammation of membranes lining the joints. Primarily it is a systemic disease, often widespread and involving many organs in its effects. Rheumatoid arthritis causes changes in joint, often bone and connective (collagen) tissue. Collagen is an elastic or semihard tissue which forms the framework supporting organs and other tissues; it is found in most places of the body. Collagen, unlike bone, is elastic.

Rheumatoid arthritis should not be self-treated because of both its variety of effects and its serious nature. Except for aspirin to relieve pain and inflammation—an important but only a small part of the treatment of rheumatoid arthritis—no over-the-counter drugs without prescription are available to treat it.

Rheumatic fever is an acute inflammation involving joints, tissues, and frequently the heart, probably due to infection, and it often follows a sore throat. Children are particularly susceptible to it. Rheumatic fever should not be self-treated.

Osteoarthritis is the arthritis that can be self-treated to reduce pain. It is a degeneration of cartilage (a form of connective tissue, gristle) and often is accompanied by a thickening or an overgrowth of bone. In contradistinction to both rheumatoid arthritis and rheumatic fever, it is not a systemic disease and has few if any direct systemic symptoms.

Fibrositis is not a joint disease at all but an inflammation of fibrous tissue such as muscle and tendon. This condition is often commonly referred to as arthritis or rheumatism, which it is not. It is also called muscular rheumatism. It is an extremely common condition and one for which over-the-counter remedies are available without prescription.

CAUSES

Merely because a chain of circumstances, happenings, or a single event precede a given condition, it does not mean that these circumstances or events have caused it.

For example, exposure to cold or emotional stress may precede rheumatoid arthritis; it may have precipitated an episode but was not the basic cause of it. The cause of rheumatoid arthritis is not known. The immediate cause of rheumatic fever is a streptococcal infection, but why some people get it and others do not, following a streptococcal infection, is not known. More profound constitutional factors may be at the root of it, in which natural resistance or other tissue conditions are at work.

The cause of osteoarthritis is essentially a breakdown of cartilage, due probably to the wear and tear of elastic tissues and joints over the years, and possibly increased by trauma. But the basic cause is less understood. Since it is not usually found in young people, but is almost universally experienced by man and other animals as he ages, there is reason to believe that that is the price man pays for aging. Osteoarthritis is not brought on by the usual stressor agents—exposure to cold, dampness, or emotional stress.

The cause of fibrositis, a common form of rheumatism—though it is not rheumatism—is uncertain, but it is believed to be precipitated by emotional stress, exposure to cold, bacterial or viral infections, trauma, perhaps stressful posture, or local tissue inflammation (which really is not a cause but a description). An epidemic form is known to be due to an infection with a specific virus.

DISCUSSION AND CAUTIONS

We shall mention *rheumatoid arthritis* only briefly, principally to differentiate it from osteoarthritis, for which over-the-counter drugs are available. Rheumatoid arthritis is also known as proliferative, atrophic, or infectious arthritis, or deformans arthritis. (See how the synonyms differ from those of osteoarthritis.) While one of the principal manifestations of rheumatoid arthritis is joint pain, it can just as well be called collagen tissue inflammation because its effects are or can be systemically widespread in the body. There are several collagen diseases, all of which are serious entities. Rheumatoid arthritis requires the service of a physician for treatment. The problems the physician has in its treatment include prevention of deformities, the treatment of complications if they arise, and devising nutritional and mechanical support, as well as physical therapy for the patient. While aspirin is often administered for pain relief, other drugs are often imperative in the treatment of rheumatoid arthritis—*none* of which are available without a prescription. Much the same situation obtains in *rheumatic fever,* with treatment perhaps at an accelerated pace, and for which no over-the-counter drugs are available. Both diseases can cripple an individual.

Osteoarthritis is a different matter. The layman has available over-the-counter drugs without prescription for the mitigation of his symptoms.

When one speaks of arthritis and rheumatism one speaks of pain. Pain is a real phenomenon. But what man *feels* cannot be expressed or evaluated without the constellations of other feelings, emotions, experiences, even fears, all of which modify his pain and characterize its existence.

All of these feelings affect an individual's *response* to pain, hence his reaction to pain. The American Indian and the Greek Spartan were culturally indoctrinated against pain; hence they responded to it least and probably with less discomfort. Western man, by and large, except in particular instances, is more responsive to pain, hence quickly takes steps to ameliorate it. In fact, in his culture it would be bizarre or masochistic for him to feel pain and do nothing about it. There are also people so highly motivated and intensely absorbed in other endeavors that their threshold of pain is higher, and they respond less to it.

Pain has concomitant events. One reaction to pain is spasm, triggered by the psyche or the nervous system. Hence, where there is pain there is often spasm. When there are pain and spasm there is also apprehension. This triad has sufficient force to accentuate the discomfort that the pain alone would produce, if one could measure it in a disembodied framework.

In osteoarthritis there is pain. It varies in intensity, depending on a person's motility or activity, his mental cast or his psychological sensitiveness, the degree of degeneration to which osteoarthritis is due, and perhaps age, for there is a positive correlation of degree of osteoarthritis and age.

Osteoarthritis is also known as degenerative joint disease and hypertrophic or degenerative arthritis. The elastic tissue becomes less elastic and thicker; hence there is pain on movement. There are also joint pain and stiffness, and later more pronounced joint changes occur with increasing discomfort. There are probably less pain and crippling than in rheumatoid arthritis, and unlike rheumatoid arthritis, there is no "hot joint" nor redness in osteoarthritis though there may be an enlargement of the joints, especially finger joints (Heberden's nodes). There are no systemic symptoms, i.e., no fever, loss of weight, etc. Pain in osteoarthritis may be in the joints that bear the weight of the body, as in the hips and knees. Pain may also occur in other places where joints are involved, as the small of the back, shoulders, or the back of the neck.

Osteoarthritis is an ancient disease. Its signs have been found in the skeletons of prehistoric animals and ancient man.

Fibrositis is probably the most common rheumatic complaint, often called muscular rheumatism. It is not rheumatism since it does not affect the joints, but does affect muscles, sheaths, tendons, or ligaments. It produces pain or soreness, and is usually associated with inflammation and stiffness.

Fibrositis does not occur in joints but in muscle anywhere in the body—lower back, etc. (Myositis is similar, in that it is an inflammation of voluntary muscles, particularly of the locomotor system.)

Fibrositis is often associated with systemic symptoms, notably fatigue. The best description for fibrositis is muscle pain. It is probably more frequent than osteoarthritis because it occurs at any age, and is usually ascribed to overexertion, "cold in the muscles." In fact, it may be the painful concomitant of the common cold, where "aching all over" is a usual complaint.

INGREDIENTS

No products used in the treatment of rheumatoid arthritis or rheumatic fever are described here because these conditions should not be self-medicated.

However, the discomforts of osteoarthritis can be ameliorated by products available over-the-counter without prescription. To supplement these, several measures are necessary.

The first is a program of rest and exercise. Rest overcomes the pain on movement, and controlled exercise extends mobility. A physician usually prescribes how much and what kind of each is desirable, because the need for each differs among individuals.

A second need is to reduce body weight, if the individual is overweight, to lighten the load on the affected joints. Considerably overweight people often find that measure alone can reduce the intensity of the pain.

However, analgesics may be necessary. Aspirin or one of the various APC (aspirin-phenacetin-caffeine) preparations is available and serves the purpose of ameliorating the pain of osteoarthritis. (See also under *Headache.*) It treats that symptom—pain—but it does nothing toward curing or even improving the basic condition itself. In fact, no drugs are known that cause a regression of the changes in joints and elastic tissue which are probably the cause of osteoarthritis.

In osteoarthritis, phenacetin and acetaminophen are as

reasonable to use as aspirin. Various mixtures, containing about 5 to 6 grains per tablet of one or more of the following, are easily obtained, aspirin, acetphenetidin (phenacetin), acetaminophen, salicylamide. Buffered aspirin tablets, each containing 5 grains aspirin with aluminum-magnesium buffering agent, are also suitable. And, of course, the oldest and probably the most used is aspirin in 5 grain tablets. These may be taken up to 8 or 10 tablets daily.

Buffered aspirin or buffered APC-type combinations are said to be the answer to *rapid* pain relief. They are picked up by the bloodstream—absorbed—more rapidly, on the basis of many reports. Assuming that more rapid absorption into the bloodstream means more rapid pain relief (as with effervescent aspirin preparations), it also means that the relief is not as long-lasting as when the absorption is less rapid. Buffered aspirin preparations do, however, reduce stomach irritation that may occur from aspirin. The parallel of taking aspirin—or any drug—on an empty stomach versus right after a meal when the stomach is full may be made. When a drug is taken on an empty stomach it may be more rapidly absorbed but there is therewith a greater likelihood of irritation than if the drug were taken on a full stomach, where the mixing with stomach contents dilutes the effect of contact between stomach and drug. (See also discussion under *The Common Cold.*)

However, it should be borne in mind that people who have a history of allergy or asthma may be sensitive to aspirin whether it is buffered or not; when taking it they may have an asthmatic attack or they may break out in hives. Also, when taking anticoagulants, the clotting quality of blood may be much impeded by the combination of anticoagulant and aspirin. Then too, stomach ulcer may be aggravated by aspirin, possibly less so by buffered aspirin, with less likelihood of irritation when taken with a tablespoon of antacid.

So people with aspirin sensitivity or stomach ulcer will be better served by an analgesic containing a combination of acetaminophen, salicylamide, and possibly phenacetin.

While tablets containing the above ingredients labeled to

be useful for the common cold are as suitable to take in treating the symptoms of osteoarthritis, be sure that such tablets do not contain nasal decongestants or antihistamines because they serve no purpose in ameliorating the pain and discomfort of osteoarthritis.

Products for the relief of the "muscular pains and aches" of fibrositis are the same as for osteoarthritis above, with one exception. Aspirin or buffered aspirin is most suitable, followed by salicylamide. The reason is that fibrositis, associated with colds or due to muscular overexertion, is associated with inflammation. Whereas aspirin and salicylamide are analgesic, antipyretic, and antiinflammatory, acetaminophen and phenacetin are analgesic but do not have the antiinflammatory effect that is desirable in fibrositis. In the event that sensitivity to aspirin exists, or anticoagulants are currently taken, or there is a history of stomach ulcer, salicylamide is a suitable replacement for aspirin.

In fibrositis, an additional agent may be used—an external analgesic rub. For information on these products, see *Muscle Pain.*

If Your Need Is for a Product Against Rheumatism (Osteoarthritis):

Look for Products Containing the Following Ingredients:

Aspirin (buffered or unbuffered)
APC tablets
Acetaminophen
Salicylamide

(In fibrositis, aspirin or salicylamide is preferable due to antiinflammatory effect.)

(Note that treatment of osteoarthritis includes a program of rest and exercise, reduction of body weight, and other measures. Analgesics supply only part of the need—to ameliorate pain.)

Avoid the Following Ingredients:

People who are sensitive to aspirin or who are taking anticoagulants should avoid aspirin, as well as aspirin-containing drugs, such as APC tablets. Those with stomach ulcer should take aspirin cautiously, as discussed in the text, if at all.

NAMES OF PRODUCTS

AGAINST ARTHRITIS AND RHEUMATISM

Anacin Tablets (Whitehall) —Contains aspirin and caffeine.

Anacin Arthritis Pain Formula (Whitehall) —Contains aspirin 7½ gr. and aluminum-magnesium buffers.

Aspirin Tablets (Various Manufacturers) —Contains aspirin 5 gr.

Bayer Timed-Release Aspirin Tablets (Bayer) —Contains aspirin 10 grains.

Bufferin Tablets (Bristol-Myers) —Contains aspirin 5 gr., with aluminum-magnesium buffers.

Empirin Compound (Burroughs Wellcome) —Contains phenacetin 2½ gr., aspirin 3½ gr., and caffeine ½ gr.

Excedrin Tablets (Bristol-Myers) —Contains acetaminophen 1½ gr., salicylamide 2 gr., aspirin 3 gr., and caffeine 1 gr.

Measurin Timed-Release Aspirin Tablets (Glenbrook) —Contains 10 gr. aspirin.

Nebs Tablets (Eaton) —Contains acetaminophen 325 mg. (5 gr.).

Tylenol Tablets (McNeil) —Contains acetaminophen 325 mg. (5 gr.).

Valadol Tablets (Squibb) —Contains acetaminophen 325 mg. (5 gr.).

MUSCLE PAIN

DEFINITION

Muscle discomfort is a sensation ranging from a slight soreness to actual pain, usually felt in twinges upon movement or without movement. While these sensations may be felt in muscle or tendon, a feeling of tightness may be due to painlike sensation in the skin itself.

CAUSES

Overexertion, especially in unaccustomed exercise and sports using muscles not normally used to that extent, bacterial or viral infections such as the common cold or influenza, and trauma are among the many possible reasons for muscle soreness or muscle pain. However, muscle pain can also be associated with trichinosis and other serious infections, impediments to circulation, diseases of metabolic origin, neurological disease, etc. Since drugs for the latter conditions are not available over-the-counter without prescription, they will not be considered here.

DISCUSSION AND CAUTIONS

Liniments are the prototype preparations used externally to mitigate or treat muscle discomfort. Balms and ointments, also used for the same purpose, usually have the same ingredients, and differ from liniments only by being in semisolid form while liniments are liquids. *Embrocation* is an old synonym for liniment. All these preparations together are called rubefacients (literally, *to make red*).

All of the rubefacients are irritants to the skin, which is the quality desired. Local irritation brings blood near the surface of the skin by dilating the small blood vessels, thus warming, hence lending a sense of comfort to the area. Often, liniments have a deeper analgesic effect than merely a local effect, without necessarily being absorbed except superficially. Deep absorption of rubefacients is not necessary. The feeling of warmth is brought on by the effect of liniments on blood vessels—it dilates them.

The heat engendered by the rubefacients is highly useful in pain relief, particularly that due to muscle pain. Thus these agents are useful in fibrositis (muscular rheumatism) and myositis and when there is muscle pain in osteoarthritis. But liniments do not cure osteoarthritis.

Heat in the form of an electric heating pad can probably serve the same purpose. The effect, however, is not as intense, as there is much less irritation experienced. Hence, there is less chance of pain relief through reflex action. Moreover, some of the rubefacient agents are absorbed through the unbroken skin, as methyl salicylate (artificial oil of wintergreen), which appears in the urine after use on the skin. It has an analgesic action similar to salicylates or aspirin.

These agents are also useful as a rubdown after vigorous exertion. Mixtures of methyl salicylate and alcohol as a rubdown after athletic exercise are old examples of another salubrious use to which these substances are put.

While these externally applied agents have their considerable usefulness, there are conditions in which they should be used with caution—or should not be used at all. One of them is a circulatory deficit.

With increasing age and its attendant arteriosclerosis there is often a restriction of circulation in the leg. There is pain on walking, relieved by stopping. The condition is called intermittent claudication, which does not really say much, because *intermittent* means recurrent and *claudication* means a limp. The condition characterized by limp or pain on walking, which ceases upon stopping, is due to a reduced or restricted circulation of the leg. In such a condition there is obviously less blood going through the leg, creating an oxygen deficit because blood brings oxygen to the tissues. Rubefacients should not be used when there is severely restricted circulation in the legs.

Another caution should be observed when using liniments: the site of application should not be bandaged, as the skin may blister.

Everyone knows, of course, not to bring these preparations in contact with the eyes. But does everyone remember to wash hands with hot soapy water after having used a liniment, on oneself or others? When eyes are touched or rubbed with the residue of liniment on hands, acute eye irritations can occur.

INGREDIENTS

There are numerous local irritants used as liniments.

Methyl salicylate or oil of wintergreen is the substance probably used more often than others. It is absorbed by the unbroken skin and has analgesic as well as irritant properties. It usually comprises 5% to 30% of a liniment. It is poisonous if swallowed; because of its pleasant odor (to some people) it may entice children and it should be kept out of their reach. Salicylate poisoning, due to aspirin or methyl salicylate, adds a substantial proportion to annual cases of poisoning.

Menthol, camphor, thymol, and eucalyptol are next in popularity as liniment ingredients. Menthol is irritating, cooling and slightly analgesic. Camphor is a somewhat more pronounced local analgesic; eucalyptol is merely irritating, which is the case with most volatile oils; thymol is antiseptic and a mild local anesthetic. The combination of menthol and camphor as ingredients in liniments is perhaps the most useful one of the above ingredients, after methyl salicylate.

Turpentine, the irritating ingredient of white liniment, is a reasonably good irritant and, when mixed with olive or sesame oil or as an emulsion with water, is a useful liniment that serves its purpose and does not usually blister, if not bandaged. But some people are hypersensitive to it.

Other rubefacients: capsicum is an oleoresin of red pepper; allyl isothiocyanate is an artificial volatile oil of mustard, effective but more likely to burn or blister unless used in a proportion of not more than 1%; chloroform and chloral—better rubefacients than these two are available; alcohol or isopropyl alcohol—used as a solvent, base, diluent or rubefacient and is satisfactory; methacholine chloride and histamine dihydrochloride are drastic counterirritants—effective but may produce blisters or wheals unless used in only small proportions, not more than about 0.25%.

Hot water bottles or electric heating pads are also used to bring local heat. They have the disadvantage of not conferring a strong or continuous feeling of warmth. Hot water bottles cool too quickly. Electric heating pads are usually not hot enough.

For that reason, some people fill hot water bottles with hot salt water (brine) or hot sugar syrup to make hot water bottles hotter. It is true that brine and syrup have a higher boiling point than water.

But *don't* do it! If the bottle breaks you will be scalded. You can also be scalded by very hot water if the bottle breaks.

Boiled water is too hot to apply to the skin. And in using a heating pad be sure that it does not become wet, through perspiration or liquid spilling on it. If the pad gets wet you may get quite a shock.

There are comparatively few occasions to use liniments on children. For the occasional use, in small quantities, liniments may serve a good purpose. Children at times develop aches and pains which parents may call "growing pains." *There are no growing pains.* Unfortunately, what are considered growing pains may possibly be prodromal signs of rheumatic fever! If the muscle pain is accompanied by hot, swollen joints or is present for more than a few days, do not use liniments but consult your physician!

If Your Need Is for a Product Against Muscle Pain:

Look for Liniments Containing the Following Ingredients:
- Oil of wintergreen
- Menthol, camphor, thymol, or eucalyptol
- Turpentine

Avoid overirritation with liniments.

NAMES OF PRODUCTS

LINIMENTS

Absorbine Arthritic Pain Lotion (Young)—Contains methyl salicylate, methyl nicotinate, and menthol.

Banalg Liniment (Cole)—Contains menthol, camphor, methyl salicylate, and eucalyptus oil in a nongreasy base.

Ben Gay (Pfizer)—Contains methyl salicylate, menthol, and lanolin.

Ben Gay Children's Ointment (Pfizer)—Contains methyl salicylate, menthol, and lanolin.

Ben Gay Pain Relieving Lotion (Pfizer)—Contains methyl salicylate, menthol, and lanolin.

(Above three products may differ only in proportion of active ingredients, which are not stated.)

Capsolin Ointment (Parke, Davis)—Contains capsicum, camphor, oil of turpentine, and oil of cajeput.

Counterpain Rub (Squibb)—Contains methyl salicylate, eugenol, and menthol.

Heet Liniment (Whitehall)—Contains capsicum, chloroform, methyl salicylate, camphor, and alcohol 53%.

Menthofax Ointment (Burroughs Wellcome)—Contains methyl salicylate 40%, menthol 6%, eucalyptol 3%, and camphor 1%.

Mentholatum Ointment (Mentholatum Co.)—Contains menthol, camphor, boric acid, and aromatic oils.

Minard's Liniment (Minard)—Contains turpentine, ammonia water, camphor, and ammonium chloride.

Minit-Rub Ointment (Bristol-Myers)—Contains camphor, menthol, oil of eucalyptus, methyl salicylate, and lanolin.

Omega Oil (Block Drug)—Contains methyl salicylate, chloroform 12%, capsicum, methyl nicotinate, histamine dihydrochloride, and isopropyl alcohol 48%.

Sloan's Liniment (Warner-Lambert)—Contains capsicum, methyl salicylate, turpentine, oils of camphor and pine.

EYE, EAR, NOSE, THROAT— AND MOUTH

DISCUSSION AND CAUTIONS

"The eyes are the mirror of the soul" is an old metaphoric saying. Few take it literally. Yet, it is a fact that many diseases of the body are mirrored in the eyes, in the mouth, in the throat. Even the skin reflects certain disease conditions of the body. Hence, the problem in a sore throat may lie anywhere in the body and may be merely manifested in the throat, or the eyes, or even the mouth.

For that reason it should be remembered that some discomforts of the eyes, ears, nose, and throat or mouth may not be local, merely the signal of the disturbance is local. And for the same reason many eye-ear-nose-throat preparations which have been available over-the-counter without prescription are now justifiably sold on prescription only. This applies to certain ear drops particularly. If relief is not obtained in a very few days with an over-the-counter product, consult a physician.

EYE

Some dysfunctions of the eye, such as jerking of the eyeballs (nystagmus), may be due to disturbances of the central nervous system or of the neuromuscular apparatus that controls the eyeballs. Drops do not strengthen eye muscles. The eye is also subject to infections. Some simple ones respond to washing with warm water. Other infections, such as those with *Pseudomonas* organisms, are most serious and in grave instances can lead to loss of vision.

Even an inflammation of the mucous membrane of the eyelids, conjunctivitis, may be the result of a systemic viral or bacterial infection, such as measles, pneumonia, or herpes. Other cases of conjunctivitis are associated with a cold and improve as the cold improves.

However, the usual complaint about eyes is irritation. This may be due to exposure to smoke, eyestrain such as working under poor light, or simply particulate matter which gets into the eyes on windy days. The eyes not only feel "tired" and have other discomforts, but are bloodshot.

For these conditions eye drops which are available over-the-counter without prescription serve satisfactorily. They usually work after several drops have been instilled into the eyes, and by reducing the bloodshot appearance may lend a refreshed feeling to the eyes and seem to bring a *bright* look and to soothe. Eye washes, using an eyecupful to wash the eye, are also available; they are refreshing, cleansing, cooling, and comforting for minor irritations but they are not as effective as eye drops. The reason is that many eye drops contain astringents, as ephedrine or zinc sulfate, which are vasoconstrictors.

INGREDIENTS

When using eye drops, choose one that contains small quantities, about 0.1%, of ephedrine and zinc sulfate. Ephedrine hydrochloride (or sulfate), the same as in nasal decongestants, is a vasoconstrictor and constricts the tiny blood vessels, which accounts for the clearing effect on bloodshot eyes. Zinc sulfate, an astringent, also constricts. Tetrahydrozoline hydrochloride (Tyzine) is similar to ephedrine, both chemically and pharmacologically, but ephedrine is used more widely. Phenylephrine hydrochloride (Neo-Synephrine) and naphazoline (Privine), also used in nasal decongestants, are similar to ephedrine and are also used in eye drops.

Note, however, that the proportions of ephedrine, tetrahydrozoline, phenylephrine, naphazoline—all hydrochlorides —when used in nose drops as nasal decongestants are in a much higher strength than in eye drops. Therefore, do not use nasal decongestants in the eye. Moreover, eye drops are sterile; nasal decongestants do not long remain sterile. Antipyrine is a slight analgesic and may lend a slight vasoconstrictive effect, but ephedrine is clearly superior.

Other ingredients used in eye drops or eye washes may serve other purposes. Thimerosal (Merthiolate), chlorobutanol, benzalkonium chloride (Zephiran), are germicides and are included to keep the eye drop solutions sterile; ethylenediaminetetraacetic acid (EDTA), a chelating agent, keeps the solution clear.

Additional ingredients are much less important, but they have been used traditionally to keep acidity and alkalinity, or to keep the solution isotonic so that it does not sting, or to prevent the solution from molding. These are boric acid (not reliable), borax (sodium borate), witch hazel, sodium or potassium chloride, or camphor water. Some contain hydrastine or berberine hydrochloride—of dubious value, but they have been traditionally used.

By and large, eye washes (in contradistinction to eye drops) are merely more dilute solutions.

If Your Need Is for a Product Against Simple Irritation of the Eye:

Look for Products Containing the Following Ingredients:

- Ephedrine
- Zinc sulfate
- Boric acid

Avoid contaminating eye drops. They are sterile when packed. Do not touch dropper to eyelid.

NAMES OF PRODUCTS

EYE DROPS

Aziza Medicated Eye Drops (Prince Matchabelli)—Contains phenylephrine hydrochloride and zinc sulfate in a water solution.

Collyrium Eye Drops (Wyeth)—Contains boric acid, borax, antipyrine, ephedrine, and thimerosal.

Eye-Gene (Pearson)—Contains phenylephrine hydrochloride, boric acid, borax, salt, sodium bisulfate, camphor water, peppermint water, and thimerosal.

Murine (Abbott)—Contains potassium bicarbonate, potassium borate, berberine hydrochloride, boric acid, glycerine, hyrastine hydrochloride, benzalkonium chloride, and thimerosal.

Ocusol Eye Drops (Norwich)—Contains boric acid, borax, salt, rose water, camphor water, witch hazel, glycerine, ephedrine hydrochloride, and thimerosal.

Visine (Leeming/Pacquin)—Contains tetrahydrozoline hydrochloride, boric acid, borax, salt, sodium ethylenediaminetetraacetate, and benzalkonium chloride.

Zincfrin Eye Drops (Alcon)—Contains zinc sulphate ¼% and phenylephrine hydrochloride 0.12%.

20/20 Eye Drops (SSS Company)—Contains boric acid, potassium chloride, zinc sulfate, naphazoline hydrochloride, camphor water, and thimerosal.

EYE WASHES

Collyrium Eye Lotion (Wyeth)—Contains antipyrine, boric acid, borax, and thimerosal.

Lavoptik (Lavoptik)—Contains boric acid, camphor, sodium chloride, hydrastine hydrochloride, and benzalkonium chloride.

Ocusol Eye Lotion (Norwich)—Contains boric acid, salt, borax, phenylephrine hydrochloride, benzalkonium chloride, and berberine hydrochloride.

EAR

The old adage says that the safest thing that can be inserted into the ear is the elbow. And when a need for an ear drop arises because of pain, an elbow may well be the safest item to insert. The reason is that pain and inflammation of the ear, which are the symptoms for which ear drops are usually sought, may be signs of a serious condition that should have the attention of a physician. It is with good reason that no ear drops, except those used to soften ear wax, are now available over-the-counter without a prescription.

Ear infections may lead to deafness which can come from inflammation of the middle ear (otitis media). There are several types of organisms that may produce such infections; those with *Proteus* or *Pseudomonas* organisms may be persistent and serious. Discomfort in the ear through changes in atmospheric pressure, as from diving or riding in an airplane, usually subsides when the individual is out of the water or the airplane lands. Sometimes the eustachian tube is blocked and needs to be blown clear by a physician. Occasionally, holding a nostril and swallowing may relieve it.

The only condition for which ear drops may be used—and in fact, the only ones available over-the-counter without prescription—are those that soften ear wax. Impacted wax may produce a cough by reflex action or may cloud hearing or produce noises.

INGREDIENTS

Ear wax is softened by warm (not hot) glycerine, by urea in glycerine, or by propylene glycol. Several drops are instilled into the ear canal, or it may be filled with the drops, allowed to remain for one-half to one hour (the patient should sit quietly during this time), and gently syringed out with warm water at body temperature, while the head is inclined to the side on which this is done. The objective is to let the water run out of the ear by gravity. But if any inflammation, heat or redness is present, such drops should not be used. They may create damage or, in fact, may delay adequate attention to the ear.

If Your Need Is for a Product for the Removal of Ear Wax:

Look for Products Containing the Following Ingredients (for removal of wax only):

Urea
Glycerine
Peroxide

Avoid everything else.

NAMES OF PRODUCTS

EAR DROPS

Debrox Ear Drops (International Pharmaceutical)—Contains carbamide (urea), peroxide, and glycerine.

Kerid Ear Drops (Blair Labs.)—Contains urea, glycerine, propylene glycol with chlorobutanol.

NOSE

The over-the-counter products available without prescription to be used in the nostrils are usually decongestants, to shrink the engorged mucous membrane of the nostrils, in order to ease breathing. These products are described under *The Common Cold* in the section on nasal decongestants.

However, at times nose drops are sought for other conditions. Among these are loss of sense of smell or distortion of smell. If they are not due to a sinus infection or do not occur during a cold, when the nasal passage is obstructed and the sense of smell is greatly reduced or temporarily lost, these are serious conditions requiring expert advice. A distortion of smell or loss of sense of smell may originate in the nervous system. It may be due to injury to a nerve by trauma or by a new growth (tumor).

In no other condition, except as indicated in the symptoms of cold and hay fever, should nose drops be used. (For names of products, see *The Common Cold.*)

If Your Need Is for a Product Against Stuffy Nose:

(See table on pages 47–48 under *Decongestants.*)

THROAT

A sore throat is often associated with a cold, during which there is pain on swallowing associated with inflamed tonsils (tonsillitis), inflammation or discomfort in the area in the back of the throat (pharyngitis) or lower in the throat, i.e., the larynx (laryngitis). These conditions are considered to be minor discomforts which leave when the cold disappears. (See *The Common Cold.*)

However, the throat is an extraordinary organ, in which serious and far-reaching diseases manifest themselves. In this respect it is probably only second to the mouth. For example, long-continued laryngitis may be due to cancer of the larynx. A sore throat is often one of the early signs of infectious mononucleosis or other infections, such as the viral Coxsackie A disease. Also, infection with the dread beta hemolytic streptococcus is most serious; it is the infecting organism in strep throat which can lead to rheumatic fever or kidney damage, if not treated.

For these conditions antibiotics are prescribed by a physician. Note should be taken that the persistent sore throat may be a streptococcal infection that should have medical attention—and don't use a cough mixture—to prevent an extension of a potentially infectious process.

INGREDIENTS

Throat *troches* are little tablets containing medication which are kept in the mouth to dissolve slowly and supply a continuous source of medication. For all practical purposes, a throat *lozenge* is the same—originally it was called a lozenge because it was diamond-shaped. Most of the troches contain an antiseptic or germicide; and some also contain menthol or peppermint to improve the taste and lend a cooling sensation; others contain benzocaine, a local anesthetic to reduce the tickle or irritation of a sore throat. The antiseptic ingredients are commonly the same as in mouthwashes (page 138). A preferable type of troche contains a germicide and benzocaine, which is a local anesthetic, though some people find the sensation of slight local anesthesia unpleasant.

While the germicides in troches are usually the same as in

mouthwashes, there is a considerable difference in their usage: a mouthwash is in contact with the mucous membrane of the mouth or throat for a very short time—a minute or two—and the remainder is quickly diluted. Therefore, there is only a rare instance of irritation with a mouthwash, unless a user happens to be sensitive to a particular substance.

However, a troche is in continuous contact with the mucous membrances of the mouth and throat. For that reason, while some people may not have irritation from a mouthwash, some may find a troche containing the same ingredients to be irritating. In that case, changing to another brand, containing a different germicide, may often solve the problem.

Troches offer a better means of treating throat irritation than gargles, because gargles just do not reach. In the process of gargling, the throat constricts and prevents contact between gargle and lower throat tissue.

The following ingredients are *antiseptic,* some with detergent effect:

cetyldimethylbenzylammonium chloride
phenol
cetylpyridinium chloride
menthol
dequalinium chloride
thymol
phenylmercuric nitrate

A local anesthetic is benzocaine.

If Your Need Is for a Product Against Throat Irritation:

Look for Lozenges Containing the Following Ingredients:
Cetyldimethylbenzylammonium chloride
Cetylpyridinium chloride
Benzocaine
Phenylmercuric nitrate
Hexachlorophene
Hexylresorcinol

NAMES OF PRODUCTS

THROAT LOZENGES

Aspergum (Pharmaco)—Consists of aspirin.

Cepacol Anesthetic Troches (Merrell)—Contains benzocaine and Ceepryn (cetylpyridinium chloride).

Chloraseptic Lozenges (Eaton)—Contains phenol, menthol, and thymol.

Isodettes Antibacterial Throat Lozenges (Isodine Pharmacal)—Contains cetyldimethylbenzylammonium chloride and benzocaine.

Lactona Anesthetic Lozenges (Warner-Lambert)—Contains benzocaine.

Listerine Throat Lozenges (Warner-Lambert)—Contains hexachlorophene. Different flavors. Children's variety contains 2.4 mg. hexachlorophene.

Lozilles Lozenges (White)—Contains propyl-*p*-aminobenzoate (an anesthetic).

Medicated Throat Discs (Parke, Davis)—Contains chloroform, capsicum, peppermint, anise, cubeb, licorice, and linseed.

Meggazones (Heggeson)—Contains menthol, peppermint, benzoin, and chloroform.

Micrin Antibacterial Throat Lozenges (Johnson & Johnson)—Contains cetylpyridinium chloride, dequalinium chloride, and benzocaine.

Phe-Mer-Nite Throat Tablets (Massengill)—Contains phenylmercuric nitrate (an excellent germicide) and benzocaine.

Smith Brothers Medicated Cough Drops (Warner-Lambert)—Contains benzocaine, menthol, and eucalyptol.

Spec-T Antibacterial Troches for Sore Throat (Squibb)—Contains cetylpyridinium chloride and benzocaine.

Spec-T Troches, Sore Throat Decongestant (Squibb)—Contains benzocaine, phenylephrine hydrochloride, and phenylpropanolamine hydrochloride.

Sucrets Sore Throat Lozenges (Quinton/Merck)—Contains hexylresorcinol. (There are several varieties of Sucrets Throat Lozenges.)

Sucrets Sore Throat Spray (Quinton/Merck)—Contains benzocaine and alcohol 34%.

Thantis Lozenges (Hynson, Westcott & Dunning)—Contains Merodicein 1/8 gr. (topical antiseptic) and saligenin 1 gr. (topical anesthetic).

Vicks Medi-Trating Throat Lozenges (Vick)—Contains benzocaine, camphor, menthol, eucalyptus oil, and cetylpyridinium chloride.

MOUTH

If the eyes are the windows of the soul, the mouth is the hall of mirrors, reflecting a great variety of disease conditions. In fact, lesions in the mouth are often used to help or to confirm diagnosis when a disease is suspected. For example, certain white, pinhead-size spots on a red patch, found on the inside of the cheeks and the inside of the lower lip—called Koplik's spots—appear before a skin rash or other signs of measles appear. In that way these spots are an early diagnostic aid. A smooth, red tongue which is suggestive of pernicious anemia, mouth ulcers which often accompany other forms of anemia, the black line on the gums in cases of chronic poisoning by lead or mercury, the dark spots inside of the cheek or tongue in Addison's disease, are other diagnostic aids.

Nutritional diseases, especially deprivation of the B vitamins, are reflected in characteristic signs on the tongue and lips. Certain skin diseases also show signs in the mouth. In one, called exudative multiform erythema, in which there are signs in eyes, throat and skin, there are characteristic blisters in the mouth.

The mouth is also subject to fungous infections, one of which is thrush. This is an infection by a fungus, *Candida albicans,* which can also affect the vagina or other mucous membranes. An antifungal material, available only on prescription, is used for this disease. None of these conditions should be self-treated.

A simpler condition, called canker sores (aphthous stomatitis), is also due to infection by a virus. Alum crystals are used in its treatment and are often successful.

Many products are offered as mouthwashes and gargles.

Most, but not all of them, are germicidal. Some are merely alkaline solutions for cleansing the mouth and rinsing out debris. These are the older type solutions. The more modern ones are antiseptic and germicidal. While they "kill germs on contact" (bacteria, not viruses) the mouth does not and cannot remain sterile; in fact, it is doubtful if continuous sterility is desirable. Sterility kills the enzymes—ptyalin, for one—that start digestion of starch in the mouth. Mouthwashes may be useful for some infectious processes, but they do not kill viruses at all.

Mouthwashes do not prevent tooth decay, but they do aid mouth cleanliness, are useful for bad breath at least temporarily, but have no effect if halitosis is due to infected teeth. The mouthwashes that are germicidal are useful as a spray or gargle in sore throat, though gargling may not touch the locus of trouble. But when used before tooth extraction they may be useful. Those that contain a local anesthetic do temporarily mitigate pain of sore throat or mouth irritation. However, mouthwashes, even antiseptic ones, do not reduce the length or severity of a cold, even though they may lend some comfort. Remember that under normal use, mouthwashes do not remain long enough in the mouth to have a sustaining effect.

INGREDIENTS

The following ingredients are germicidal and some are surface-active agents as well: cetylpyridinium chloride (Ceepryn), beta-phenoxyethyldodecyldimethylammonium bromide (Domiphen), phenol (carbolic acid), benzethonium chloride (Phemerol, Hyamine 1622), hexylresorcinol (S.T. 37), povidone-iodine (Isodine), and chlorothymol.

The following ingredients are germicidal but are used in small quantities, hence may or may not make a germicidal solution: oils of eucalyptus, birch, pine, spearmint, peppermint, clove, cinnamon, also menthol, thymol, chlorothymol, cinnamaldehyde, methyl salicylate, eucalyptol, camphor, and benzoic acid.

All mouthwashes are aqueous solutions; water is the vehicle

for the active ingredients and the solvent. Alcohol is germicidal. In mouthwashes it is used primarily as a solvent in varying proportions for menthol and other similar substances, and contributes to the germicidal effect of the total solution, depending on the proportion of alcohol. For all practical purposes, the terms *antiseptic* and *germicide* are the same.

Zinc chloride or zinc sulfate in mouthwashes acts as a coagulant for mouth debris, which is disposed of by rinsing the mouth.

In comparing antiseptic effects, it should be noted that a mouthwash that is recommended to be used in diluted form (such as drops in half a glass of water) is much less likely to be germicidal than one used full strength.

If Your Need Is for a Product Against Mouth Irritation:

Look for Products Containing the Following Ingredients:

- Cetylpyridinium chloride
- Hexylresorcinol
- Benzethonium chloride
- Zinc sulfate or chloride

NAMES OF PRODUCTS

MOUTHWASHES

Alkalol (Alkalol Co.)—Contains thymol, eucalyptol, camphor, benzoin, alum, potassium chloride, sodium bicarbonate, salt, oils of birch, spearmint, pine and cinnamon, and 0.5% alcohol. Offered as an alkaline saline solution.

Astring-O-Sol (Sterling Drug)—Contains zinc chloride, myrrh, oil of wintergreen, and 70% alcohol.

Cepacol (Wm. S. Merrell)—Contains cetylpyridinium chloride (Ceepryn) and 14% alcohol.

Chloraseptic Mouthwash and Gargle (Norwich)—Contains phenol, borax, and thymol.

Colgate 100 (Colgate-Palmolive)—Contains benzethonium chloride and 17% alcohol.

Glyco-Thymoline (Kress & Owen)—Contains sodium benzoate, sodium bicarbonate, borax, sodium salicylate, eucalyptol, menthol, thymol, oils of sweet birch and pine, glycerine, and 4% alcohol. Offered as an alkaline cleansing solution.

Isodine Antiseptic (Blair Labs.) —Contains povidone-iodine, a combination of iodine with a polyvinyl product owing its effect to iodine.

Isodine Concentrate (Blair Labs.) —Contains povidone-iodine; needs dilution before use.

Lavoris (Vick) —Contains zinc chloride, cinnamaldehyde, clove oil, saccharin, and 5% alcohol.

Listerine (Warner-Lambert) —Contains thymol, eucalyptol, methyl salicylate, menthol, benzoic and boric acids, and 25% alcohol.

Micrin (Johnson & Johnson) —Contains cetylpyridinium chloride, oil of peppermint, menthol, and 15% alcohol.

Pepsodent Antiseptic (Lever Bros.) —Contains chlorothymol, boric acid, citric acid, and 26% alcohol.

Peroxide (Various Manufacturers) —Contains 3% hydrogen peroxide.

Reef Mouthwash (Warner-Lambert) —Contains cetylpyridinium chloride, menthol, methyl salicylate, and 18% alcohol.

Scope (Procter & Gamble) —Contains cetylpyridinium chloride, Domiphen bromide (beta-phenoxyethyldodecyldimethylammonium bromide), and 18% alcohol.

S.T. 37 Solution (Merck) —Contains hexylresorcinol.

FEMININE HYGIENE

DISCUSSION AND CAUTIONS

Archeologists have been able to reconstruct a view of a long-lost culture by the articles they found in its ruins. The search for martial or household articles is standard. Through them, the territorial, religious as well as the social life of these cultures has been reconstructed.

Products used for personal adornment or for other personal use reflect the daily lives of the people of a culture. Among the most valuable indicators of individuals who made up such a society are the toilet articles the women and men used to enhance their appearance. This is also an approximation of the ideal of their fantasies.

Those adornments followed what that particular culture decreed. For example, if hair-shaving instruments were found, it can be tentatively deduced that men shaved or cut their hair. To learn if women shaved their body hair, other additional artifacts are sought and studied. Another example: the average woman in Italy does not shave her underarms. In a future time, if the current culture would be unearthed, no delicate underarm razors will be found there (except perhaps those used by sophisticated foreign visitors).

Our current culture in the United States can well be called the deodorized society, among other names. To replace natural body odors with artificial fragrances has the approval of society. Perhaps that is indeed an advance over stale sweat. But the process of deodorization does not stop with the underarms. It even reaches with aerosol tentacles into the living rooms—which do not stink. It often enwraps women with an obnoxiously heavily perfumed aura, though they themselves do not have an unpleasant odor because baths or underarm deodorants have precluded that.

Now the deodorized society has assailed women in their last bastion—the vagina.

The deodorized culture has convinced women that they "offend" unless they accept the need of total deodorization. It appeals to their feminine vanity: "for-the-most-girl-part-of-you." It implies that women subject others to unspeakable odors unless they use the new total deodorant that happens to be touted.

The deodorized culture craftily ties on to new social mores and equates greater sexual freedom with increased body odor. So it implies that an integral part of the modern woman must be an aseptic vagina.

FEMININE SPRAYS

In the late 1960s an aerosol spray, to be directed against the pubic hair and outer lips of the vagina, appeared in Switzerland. There was comparatively little interest in that then-new product. When that product, the feminine spray, was introduced into the United States, it became apocalyptic. It revealed to women that they "offend"—and gave them a method of protecting against that social sin of "offending." With many means offering protection or prophylaxis, you do not have to submit proof, as long as you hit the fear button and offer a remedy.

It is interesting to note that part of the sexual attraction between man and woman (and between other animals as well) is based on odor. There is an individual odor, not at all necessarily unpleasant, that characterizes people. The odor of the he-man from the Western plains—sweat and tobacco—is considered masculine and desirable. The natural, clean odor of woman has now been proscribed, unless the nonodor is covered with a feminine spray, to be used "as frequently as you like."

The use of the feminine sprays is probably not harmful, though irritations have been reported in the medical press. They can irritate if the deodorizing task is done too efficiently —by spraying between the outer lips of the vagina. But the feminine sprays can damage a woman's self-esteem, by convincing her that if she does not use them she will "offend." The claims in behalf of the sprays ignore the fact that there is a dynamic equilibrium in the vagina, and the regular secretions will continue, though they are normally not perceptible in the course of outside daily contact. Advertising favors dependence on feminine sprays by recommending that they be used after moments of stress (better than a tranquilizer?). These products enter into the bedroom, in fact the conjugal bed, by being recommended for use before bedtime (instead of a bath?). They suggest use during menstruation, a reasonable idea, but the question of whether they are effective for that use remains in doubt. Then another question arises: a new, unaccustomed odor appears. Is it desirable in bed—or out of it?

Another form of feminine "spray" is not a spray, but a small paper towel moistened with an antiseptic liquid sealed in individual envelopes. It is used in the outer part of the vagina much as a cloth wipe. This may have an advantage in that, if there is a discharge, it may be wiped off.

An incidental point about odor: Charles Darwin held that in the matter of natural selection and survival, those animals which had well-developed and well-functioning odor glands were able to entice more females and to mate more easily and more frequently. Thus, they had a greater opportunity to pass on their own characteristics to their issue. In man, odor is still a vestigial sexual attractant.

INGREDIENTS

The principal ingredient of the feminine spray is an antiseptic or germicide. Hexachlorophene, long a useful ingredient in soaps, is the principal one. Other ingredients are odorants. Since feminine sprays are claimed to be only deodorants, they are considered by the Federal Food, Drug and Cosmetic Act to be cosmetics, not drugs. Hence they need not carry a list of their active ingredients. Another ingredient is methyl or propyl paraben, a preservative with a weak antiseptic property.

If you must choose to use a feminine spray as a ticket of admission to the deodorized society, select it merely by the odor you like. The powder spray has an advantage over the aerosol spray, in that a powder remains longer on the site sprayed. More particularly, a powder is absorbent, which is not the case with an aerosol spray. If used for spraying on the outside of the vagina, use it only infrequently, thus reducing the possibility of sensitization. On or near mucous membrane, the possibility of sensitization is greater than on unbroken skin.

NAMES OF PRODUCTS

FEMININE SPRAYS AND CLOTH WIPES

Bidette Mist (Young Drug Products)

Bidette Premoistened Vaginal Towelettes–Wipes (Young Drug Products) —Contains hexachlorophene, propyl paraben, and alcohol.

Demure (Vick Chemical Company)

FDS Feminine Hygiene Deodorant Spray (Alberto-Culver)

Feminique Feminine Cloth Wipes (Bristol-Myers)

Feminique Feminine Hygiene Spray (Bristol-Myers)

Koro Sanitary Napkin Deodorant Spray (Holland-Rantos) —Contains hexachlorophene and alcohol.

Massengill Feminine Deodorant Spray (Massengill) —Contains hexachlorophene.

My Own Hygienic Deodorant Spray-Vaginal (Emko)

My Own Towelettes Wipes (Emko) —Contains benzalkonium chloride.

Naturally Feminine Powder Spray (Johnson & Johnson)

Norform Feminine Spray (Norwich) —Contains hexachlorophene.

Pristeen Feminine Hygiene Deodorant Spray (Warner-Lambert)

Quest Deodorant Spray (Clark-Cleveland) —Offered for sanitary napkins and clothing.
Rantex Personal Cloth Wipes (Holland-Rantos) —Contains benzalkonium chloride, methyl paraben, and witch hazel.
Vespré Powder Spray (Johnson & Johnson)
Vespré Aerosol Spray (Johnson & Johnson)

DOUCHES

A more desirable form of product for feminine hygiene is the douche—long known, though in the past much overused. One of the reasons for its greater frequency of use before the advent of the *Pill* was for contraceptive purposes. The use of dilute vinegar douches or others after sexual intercourse is well known. Another use was for cleansing, after menstruation or even between menstrual periods.

Douches do reduce odor if it is there. Occasionally, they are good for cleansing in the event of a vaginal discharge. (A discharge may be due to infections that require medical attention.) Douches of plain water or salt and water do cleanse. But solutions made from the available douche powders sold over-the-counter without prescription cleanse considerably better because they remove mucous debris—though mucus is naturally found in the vagina. Most douches are mildly alkaline, thus cleansing better. Douches that are mildly acid are probably better and are often recommended by a physician. They approach the natural reaction of the vagina.

Another reason why women use douches is emotional, to have a *feeling* of personal cleanliness. It may or may not be justified. But feelings are often more important than facts.

Daily douches are to be avoided! Paradoxically, though they cleanse, they upset the natural vaginal ecology as to acidity, bacterial population, formation of mucus, and the natural elaboration of lubricating material. There is probably no detrimental result from a weekly douche. But a greater frequency than twice weekly is clearly undesirable.

INGREDIENTS

The ingredients in douches are either germicides or surface-active agents which, reducing surface tension, spread better and cleanse more efficiently. Some are both surface-active and germicidal and contain alkalies or acids, or materials like menthol or eucalyptol that confer a cooling sensation and a feeling of freshness. But if they are too concentrated, menthol or camphor can produce a feeling of heat through irritation. Usually douches contain combinations of these ingredients.

Among surface-active agents that are also germicides are the following (the full chemical names are given because those appear on the label, and therefore the consumer will have a point of reference): octylphenoxypolyethoxy ethanol, acetyldimethylpolyethoxy ethanol, polyoxyethylene nonylphenol (each represents a different Triton product), or benzalkonium chloride (Zephiran).

Surface-active agents that are not as germicidal as those above, but which enhance the effect of germicides because they spread, or penetrate folds, are dioctyl sodium sulfosuccinate, sodium edetate (EDTA), sodium lauryl sulfate, triethanolamine dodecylbenzene sulfonate.

Povidone-iodine (PVP-I) is an iodine complex and has the antiseptic effect of iodine. Oxyquinoline sulfate is also an antiseptic.

All germicides tend to reduce the bacterial population—fortunately temporarily.

Substances that react as alkalies are sodium bicarbonate, borax (sodium borate), and sodium perborate. Sodium perborate releases a small amount of oxygen and therefore is an oxidizing agent.

Those that react as acids are lactic acid and alum; much less important is boric acid.

While alkaline douches have their advantage in more efficient cleansing, acid douches better resemble the natural reaction of the vagina. The alkalinity or acidity is extremely mild; there is no strong alkaline or acid reaction, especially after dilution with water. The presence of one of the detergent-germicides is highly desirable, because they both cleanse and are mildly germicidal.

It is wise to make a douche solution about half the strength recommended on the label, because, except in extraordinary circumstances, the milder solution serves the same purpose. Moreover, the chance of irritation is reduced by that practice. The concentration can be easily increased, if needed, and usually it will not be found necessary. All douches are concentrated (liquids or powders) and must be diluted or dissolved before use.

If Your Need Is for a Douche:

Look for Products Containing the Following Ingredients:

- Benzalkonium chloride
- Lactic acid (in acid douches)
- Alum
- Sodium bicarbonate (in alkaline douches)
- Borax (in alkaline douches)

NAMES OF PRODUCTS

DOUCHES

Betadine Douche (Purdue Frederick)—Contains povidone-iodine complex, owing its antiseptic effect to iodine.

Demure (Vick Chemical Company)—Liquid containing benzalkonium chloride.

Jenéen (Norwich) Liquid containing lactic acid, sodium lactate, and octylphenoxypolyethoxy ethanol.

Koromex Douche Powder (Holland-Rantos)—Contains milk sugar, salt, lactic acid, urea, menthol, thymol, oil of eucalyptus, methyl salicylate, benzalkonium chloride, and polyoxyethylenenonylphenol.

Lorate (Standard Labs.)—Contains borax, peroxide, sodium bicarbonate, salt, soap, and menthol.

Lysette (Sterling Drug)—Liquid containing triethanolamine dodecylbenzene sulfonate.

Massengill Douche Powder (Massengill)—Contains boric acid, alum, berberine hydrochloride, salt, phenol, menthol, thymol, eucalyptol, and methyl salicylate. (The liquid Massengill douche, an entirely different formula, is preferable.)

Massengill Liquid Douche (Massengill)—Contains lactic acid, sodium lactate, and octylphenoxypolyethoxy ethanol.

Stomaseptine Douche Powder (Harcliff)—Contains sodium perborate, sodium bicarbonate, salt, borax, menthol, thymol, eucalyptol, and methyl salicylate.

Trichotine (Reed & Carnrick)—Available both as a liquid and as a powder containing sodium lauryl sulfate, sodium perborate, and borax.

V.A. Douche Powder (Norcliff)—Contains oxyquinoline citrate, boric acid, alum, and zinc sulfate.

Vagisec (Julius Schmidt)—Liquid containing polyoxyethylene nonylphenol, sodium edetate (EDTA), and dioctyl sodium sulfosuccinate.

Zonite (Chemway)—Liquid containing sodium hypochlorite and salt. Resembles the old Dakin's solution; newer products have since appeared.

INSOMNIA AND FATIGUE

INSOMNIA AND SLEEP INDUCERS

DEFINITION

Insomnia (sleeplessness) is the inability to sleep.

CAUSE

While sleeplessness may have profound causes, due to serious body dysfunction or pain, most commonly it is due to overexcitement, producing restlessness and preventing the relaxation that precedes sleep.

DISCUSSION AND CAUTIONS

We never cease to wonder at two phenomena which are two sides of the same coin: (a) naturally recurrent sleep and (b) awakening, which is perhaps a greater wonder.

Fantastically complex events take place in the body which produce the sleep-waking cycle. Many of those events which we can observe we do not fully understand.

One of the events connected with sleep is the biological rhythm by which sleep takes place and regularly recurs. Change of the rhythm—due to a change in a work shift, for example—disturbs the ability to fall asleep. The same break in the biological rhythm occurs in airplane pilots when they traverse several time zones from east to west or the reverse.

With them, it is virtually an occupational disease and is often responsible for digestive disturbances, irascibility, impotence, as well as sleeplessness (See *Clocks and Rhythms in Living Organisms*).

Another event that has to do with sleep is dreaming. It is only comparatively recently that REM (rapid eye movement) sleep has been described, during which dreaming takes place. Awakening an individual during REM sleep is much more disturbing than during non-REM sleep.

There are many other events connected with the marvellous cycle of sleep and awakening. Body functions continue during sleep but are much reduced, as if the fires are banked for the night. Perhaps the most important disorder of sleep is the inability to sleep: insomnia or sleeplessness.

And sleeplessness, too, has its several varieties.

The first type is the delay in falling asleep. The unrelaxed and concerned sleeper figuratively and literally turns and twists, becoming more anxious because he cannot fall asleep. That anxiety by itself further delays his sleep; then he falls asleep from sheer exhaustion. When such a sleeper awakens, he often does not feel as if he had adequate sleep. The expression "I slept only two hours" is a common one. The sleeper believes it, although he may have slept six hours. It merely feels like two hours. This is delayed sleep.

The second type of sleeplessness consists of awaking after having slept two or three hours. The period during which such an individual is awake is usually longer than in the case of the individual who took some time to fall asleep. This type of sleep—interrupted sleep—usually occurs in individuals who are in pain, are otherwise ill, and are beset and bedeviled with worry. He may fall asleep after daybreak, and must soon arise. The feeling of comfort and relaxation that sleep confers is not his upon arising.

A third type of sleeplessness is awaking at 4:00 or 5:00 A.M. with inability to return to sleep. Sometimes this is due to a vicious cycle: the sleeper awakens at 4:00 or 5:00 A.M., cannot resume sleep, and to make up goes to bed too early—hence, he normally would awake quite early. This type of sleeplessness is often the case in the anxiety-prone or depressed individual. He usually awakens before daybreak—the feedback of his anxiety begins his day.

What should one do for sleeplessness? The last resort should be medicines. But the last resort is at times a wise decision in order to break the cycle of sleeplessness. It is deadly easy to say that sleep comes when, at sleeping time, the mind is composed and the stresses of the day are put out of mind. It is easy to recommend, but hard to put into effect.

Other steps may help, to put the would-be sleeper's mind into a state of sleep-receptivity.

One is the traditional warm bath, not a shower. A shower tends to be stimulating because there is considerable movement in soaping and rinsing during a shower. In a bathtub, there is an opportunity to soak for 15 or 20 minutes, reading, smoking, or just doing nothing. There is need for *soaking—not soaping*. Warmth relaxes. Going to bed directly from the bath predisposes to relaxation preparatory to sleep.

Another presleep preparation is going to bed at about the same time nightly. This is a mild form of conditioning by itself, especially when combined with the usual presleep ritual, such as brushing teeth or preparing clothes for the next day.

Then, reading in bed with a strong light may be found helpful. A strong light tires the eyes but does not strain them. As to the reading material itself, get a boring book—say, a work on the hydrodynamics of the water-pistol. You may be glad to fall asleep to escape further reading of such an entrancing treatise. An additional presleep ritual is a hot drink, preferably nonalcoholic, such as cocoa, tea, or milk. Or a sandwich will do if you have not overdrawn your daily caloric quota. Food soothes.

In addition, put yourself in a comfortable aura in bed. When the weather is hot, try to arrange your bed so that you are cool. In winter, an electric blanket is often a marvelous sleep inducer; we know of no side effects from it, except electric shock, if you happen to spill a cup of tea on it.

But if you find that sleep is long in coming, or if you

awaken after a short time, it may be well to consider one of the over-the-counter sleep-inducers available without prescription, provided, of course, that you have checked with your physician and you are otherwise well but too tense to sleep.

Bear in mind, too, that if you develop a *habit* of taking a sleep-inducer you are defeating your desire to fall asleep naturally. When you find that one of the sleep-inducers helps you to sleep, take it alternate nights, then every third night, and stop. Introduce one of the sleep-inducing rituals into your sleep preparations. You may have to repeat the cycle of taking and stopping.

INGREDIENTS

The preparations for sleep-inducing available over-the-counter without prescription contain antihistamines, usually methapyrilene fumarate or hydrochloride, pyrilamine maleate, with or without scopolamine, which is a belladonnalike alkaloid derived from belladonna. These are the principal ingredients.

Antihistamines, as the name implies, are antagonists to histamine. Histamine is a substance released in the body when a material is taken into or introduced into or applied upon the body to which the body is oversensitive (hypersensitive) or intolerant. This is a true allergic reaction.

But sleeplessness has nothing to do with allergy (except for the sleeplessness due to allergic discomfort). The reason that antihistamines are used as sleep-inducers is their side effect. The principal side effect, used to advantage, is the production of drowsiness.

The drowsiness is the result of sedation. In that way antihistamines are sedatives—they can calm, and make one drowsy. Drowsiness is a drawback as a side effect when you need to be alert. But drowsiness can be an advantage when you need to fall asleep.

Some antihistamines are more sedative (drowsiness-producing) than others. A few of those are available only on prescription. But again, in the last event, it depends much on the individual reaction—how a given person responds to antihistamines. For that reason, one cannot say which antihistamine has the strongest side effect of drowsiness production. Some people fall asleep after one analgesic (with antihistamine) tablet taken to control cold symptoms; one such tablet contains 2 mg. chlorpheniramine hydrochloride, an antihistamine.

It is possible that you may find that a given preparation which contains a certain antihistamine may be without effect. Another preparation with a different antihistamine may well cause drowsiness enough to put you to sleep.

Another ingredient in the over-the-counter sleep-inducing products is scopolamine or scopolamine methyl bromide. These are alkaloids of belladonna and reduce muscle spasm, reduce stomach acidity, and are mildly, very mildly, sedative. For the purpose of sedation, scopolamine is preferable to scopolamine methyl bromide, as the latter has less of a sleep-inducing effect than plain scopolamine.

Salicylamide is another ingredient, though not one frequently met. It occasionally produces drowsiness, though not as predictably as the antihistamines. And you need larger doses of salicylamide than are found in the common sleep-inducing preparations sold over-the-counter.

The claims used in behalf of the antihistamine preparations to induce sleep—tension reduction (it comes with drowsiness), hence, some relaxation, and hopefully sleep—are fair by and large. Claims that promise change of mood, brightening the world, more efficient work performance are not true.

Some reports deny that antihistamines are useful as mild sleep-inducers. That is indeed bizarre: it is illogical to require labels on antihistamines to warn against doing work that requires alertness because they produce drowsiness, and on the other hand to deny their usefulness for sleep induction which depends on drowsiness production.

The difference between sedatives and hypnotics: it is largely a matter of degree. Sedatives can "settle" one sufficiently to help one to sleep. Hypnotics are drugs that, acting rapidly and strongly, actually put the user to sleep before he has a chance to relax and fall asleep naturally. Awakening after sleep brought on by hypnotics can be a trying experience, and it may take some hours to throw off a continued feeling of drowsiness.

If Your Need Is for a Product Against Sleeplessness:

Look for Products Containing the Following Ingredients:
- Methapyrilene
- Pyrilamine

NAMES OF PRODUCTS

SLEEP-INDUCERS

Compoz Tablets (Jeffrey Martin)—Contains scopolamine hydrobromide 0.15 mg., methapyrilene hydrochloride 15 mg., and pyrilamine maleate 10 mg.

Cope Tablets (Glenbrook)—Contains aspirin 6½ gr., methapyrilene fumarate ⅕ gr. (13 mg.), caffeine 30 mg. with aluminum magnesium buffer.

Dormin Capsules (Dormin)—Contains methapyrilene hydrochloride 25 mg.

Nytol Capsules (Block Drug)—Contains 50 mg. methapyrilene.

Nytol Tablets (Block Drug)—Contains methapyrilene hydrochloride 25 mg. and salicylamide.

Quiet World Tablets (Whitehall)—Contains acetaminophen 2½ gr., aspirin, methapyrilene hydrochloride 16.67 mg., and scopolamine hydrobromide 0.083 mg.

Sleep Capsules (Rexall)—Contains methapyrilene hydrochloride 50 mg., salicylamide 200 mg., and scopolamine aminoxide hydrobromide 0.5 mg.

Sleep Tablets (Rexall)—Contains methapyrilene hydrochloride 25 mg., sodium bromide 3 gr., potassium bromide 3 gr., and ammonium bromide 1½ gr.

Sleep-eze Tablets (Whitehall)—Contains methapyrilene hydrochloride 25 mg. and scopolamine hydrobromide 0.125 mg.

Sominex Tablets (J. B. Williams)—Contains scopolamine aminoxide hydrobromide 0.25 mg., methapyrilene hydrochloride 25 mg., and salicylamide 200 mg.

Tranquil-Aid Tablets (Thompson Medical)—Contains glyceryl guaiacolate, methapyrilene fumarate, salicylamide, and magnesium trisilicate.

FATIGUE, STIMULANTS, AND HANGOVER

DEFINITION

Fatigue is a feeling of weakness, tiredness, or "lack of energy."

CAUSE

The commonly accepted but perhaps the least frequent reason for fatigue is overwork. The most frequent cause of fatigue is probably psychological, arising from anxiety, depression, frustration, or other psychogenic causes. But fatigue may also be a sign of body disorders that arise from heart failure, muscle disease, infection, anemia, disorders of some glands as the thyroid or adrenal glands, or even low blood sugar.

DISCUSSION AND CAUTIONS

It is "normal" to feel fatigue after physical exertion such as unaccustomed labor or athletic participation. But recovery comes quickly after rest.

The person with a relatively sedentary job is often much fatigued at the end of the day. He does no physical labor, but he may expend a good deal of psychic energy in a frustrating environment, with work uninteresting to him. He is fatigued from frustration and the psychologically unrewarding activity of the day.

The housewife caring for children, running a household, washing dishes and cleaning, which seem never to be completed because the tasks have to be repeated daily, also gets fatigue. Her tiredness is a function compounded of physical activity, coping with children, confronting her husband who often returns home irascible from his confrontations at work, and her feeling of drudgery. Hers is a fatigue of physical endeavor with lack of stimulation.

The individual, in various settings, who is not necessarily exposed to frustration in his work, but whose activities are characterized by monotony—hence boredom—also becomes quickly fatigued. Enthusiasm and interest overcome fatigue, but how can you develop enthusiasm in the matrix of monotony?

Then there is the individual who is developmentally without drive. He does only what he must do and fears excess (he never heard of Oscar Wilde's *nothing succeeds like excess*) . He must lie down after some effort, not because he feels ill but because he feels fatigued. Even his sex drive tapers down earlier than that of other men. He does not dare to change his state—and in fact cannot. He remains chronically fatigued, though well. At times, such an individual is subjected to experiences that are emotionally stormy, from which he comes out emotionally and physically depleted.

And above all, there is the fatigue of neurosis. It is associated with depression or anxiety. At times such fatigue is accompanied by restlessness, in the presence of depression, complicating the picture and increasing the load on the person who bears it. All these people seek a remedy for fatigue. After a time, unfortunately, fatigue becomes a way of life.

An entirely different individual is the "success-oriented" man who desires to accentuate nature. For example, while not fatigued, except temporarily and occasionally, he feels the need to be more alert when awake, more energetic in his work and more potent in his sexual endeavors.

The desire to exceed does not necessarily make one excel. It is a cultural phenomenon, an expression of an era that puts a value on quantity rather than quality. This type of individual wants to *avoid* fatigue, so that he can continue to exceed.

Further, the student wants to avoid fatigue and stay awake while cramming for his examination. He, too, wants to avoid fatigue and be more alert when awake.

All these people are greatly concerned with fatigue—to overcome it or to prevent it.

The needs of different individuals are not the same. A single drug to dispel fatigue grossly oversimplifies the problem. If it temporarily gives a boost of energy, it does so at a price that is too high. This applies to amphetamines, not available over-the-counter. In a much smaller measure it also applies to another stimulant, caffeine. Caffeine is available over-the-counter without prescription, for certain needs, at certain times, and not for continuing or regular use.

INGREDIENTS

We do not consider it extraordinary for a person to take a cup of coffee when in need of a "lift." Yet, we look askance if he takes a tablet containing about the same amount of caffeine. This is due to our stereotypes, by which we unfortunately operate in many areas. The cry of *drug culture* is heard, whereas we already have an alcohol culture.

Caffeine is a powerful stimulant to the higher nervous centers (central nervous system). Hence, it stimulates mental activity, helps sustain it, and stimulates the free flow of the thinking process. It also reduces drowsiness and fatigue—the reason for its use by students while studying. In addition, it enhances physical activity, probably due to the fact that caffeine stimulates muscular function. In general, it "tones up" the body.

A perfect tonic? Far from it.

The negative parts: The stimulation draws on body reserves, and when it has worn off, depression often ensues. Then, an excessive amount of caffeine has extended effects; it produces sleeplessness (an extension of its alert-inducing effect) and excitement. Remember the story of the *Sorcerer's Apprentice:* do not overwind with caffeine as you may find it difficult to stop running. As a substitute for sleep it can indeed be dangerous.

Too much caffeine can give you palpitations and other heart irregularity, which can be frightening while you have them. And if you have a stomach ulcer, or a suspicion of one, do not take caffeine or coffee. Reason? It stimulates extra acidity which you do not want for stomach ulcer.

In comparing the advantages of caffeine with its detrimental effects, it appears that the judicious use of caffeine or coffee has assets: it stimulates mentally, somewhat physically, and may help cope with problems—with which we should be able to cope without coffee.

Certainly, it is not imprudent to take caffeine or have a cup of coffee if it will temporarily lift fatigue to help get a job done.

A cup of coffee contains about 100 to 125 mg. caffeine. The dose of caffeine is about 125 to 250 mg., equivalent to 1 to 2 cups of coffee.

Should you take a caffeine tablet or a cup of coffee?

Coffee is vastly better. For one thing, it also stimulates good social interaction. The American coffee break habit is equivalent to the older European practice of breaking bread with a friend or a stranger.

Incidentally, while tea contains more caffeine than coffee, the effective amount of caffeine per cup is about the same. The reason lies in the fact that less tea is used in making a cup.

Cola drinks also contain caffeine, but much less than coffee. The usual 12-ounce can or bottle contains 40 to 60 mg. caffeine.

The danger of coffee or cola drinks can be, and is, a nutritional problem. It should not be used instead of food—often the habit with teen-agers who can least afford such a substitute, as they have particular nutritional needs during growth.

The only advantages that caffeine tablets have over a cup of coffee is their portability. They can be used when coffee is unavailable. Since coffee is a hot drink, that, too, adds to the stimulating effect, another reason for its preference over caffeine tablets.

An additional product offered for fatigue is a tablet that contains analgesics with caffeine. We fail to see its usefulness unless taken for a headache. When choosing a caffeine tablet, select the one that states on the label the amount of caffeine it contains. You will then be able to equate it in terms of cups of coffee.

Another stimulant has recently appeared on the market which purports to give a much needed lift for alcoholic hangover. It contains caffeine, vitamin B_1, niacin, acetaminophen, but above all, aspirin.

Aspirin is the last thing you need in connection with or after alcoholic indulgence. The reason is that aspirin has a propensity for causing bleeding points in the stomach, and this effect is accentuated in combination with alcohol. It may make an alcoholic gastritis worse or may cause gastritis. (See discussion on aspirin under analgesics in *The Common Cold* and in *Arthritis and Rheumatism.*)

We do not recommend reliance on *any* hangover remedy even if it were found to be effective. Even if it quickly relieves an alcoholic hangover the damage of alcoholic overindulgence is done. You cannot negate the effects of destruction of both brain cells or functioning liver cells brought about by overindulgence in alcohol. The attrition continues with each binge. Another danger of alcoholic overindulgence: alcoholic habituation razes horizontally—physically, societally, economically, and spiritually.

If Your Need Is for a Product Against Fatigue:

Look for Products Containing the Following Ingredients:
  Caffeine
Avoid the Following Ingredients:
  Amphetamine or other "uppers"

NAMES OF PRODUCTS

STIMULANTS

Chaser for Hangover (Cary)—Contains acetaminophen 160 mg., caffeine 100 mg., niacinamide 10 mg., *aspirin 160 mg.,* thiamine mononitrate 25 mg., oil of peppermint, aluminum and magnesium buffers.

Comeback Tablets (Thayer)—Contains acetaminophen, salicylamide and caffeine alkaloid.

Enerjets Tablets (Chilton)—Contains caffeine.

Kirkaffeine (Moore-Kirk)—Contains 250 mg. caffeine.

Nodoz Tablets (Bristol-Myers)—Contains 100 mg. caffeine.

Tirend Tablets (Norcliff)—Contains caffeine, niacin, dextrose, and thiamine mononitrate.

Vivarin Stimulant Tablets (J. B. Williams)—Contains 200 mg. caffeine and 150 mg. dextrose.

ALLERGY

BRONCHIAL ASTHMA

DEFINITION

Bronchial asthma may be due to an allergic condition. It differs from hay fever in that the problem lies in difficulty in breathing. There is wheezing due to contraction or constriction of smaller bronchial vessels, and discomfort in the in-out breathing but especially in exhaling or breathing out. (Do not confuse it with cardiac asthma, which is a heart and lung condition also called acute pulmonary edema, in which there is also difficulty in breathing. The cause here is vastly different. Cardiac asthma is *not* an allergic disease.)

CAUSE

As an allergic condition, the cause usually lies in sensitivity (hypersensitivity) to some material. Unlike hay fever, which occurs usually in the summer or fall when a great deal of pollen is in the air, bronchial asthma is not necessarily seasonal. When the sensitive person is brought in contact with the stuff to which he is sensitive (an allergen) there is constriction of the bronchial muscles and vessels. There is difficulty in breathing or in expulsing mucus, and the typical asthma attack ensues. The triggering cause is an inhaled or ingested allergen, or infection in the respiratory tract.

DISCUSSION AND CAUTIONS

Both hay fever and bronchial asthma are allergic conditions. Not only are the symptoms different, but the disease mechanism is different. And the remedies to control it are different. For example, antihistamines, which are useful in hay fever, are of limited use in bronchial asthma. Sometimes they may be helpful in preventing an attack, but are not reliable for that purpose.

In our opinion, preparations for the use of controlling bronchial asthma should not be available without a prescription, despite the fact that they often help. At least, before they are used, the person with bronchial asthma should see his doctor to assess his condition.

There are several reasons for that. *One,* adults who have bronchial asthma do not "outgrow" it; it usually becomes worse with advancing age. *Two,* conditions such as infections somewhere in the respiratory tract, which can bring on a spell of bronchial asthma, cannot be determined or assessed by the person who has them, though he can often tell best what best relieves him. *Three,* the proportion of the ingredients in bronchial asthma preparations is often too small—as aminophylline or theophylline—to give optimum relief. *Four,* some of the effective over-the-counter products available without prescription, as epinephrine, often have certain side effects or can affect other body functions; they should first be prescribed by a physician, and subsequently they can be bought over-the-counter without prescription. *Five,* when bronchial asthma becomes chronic—after having been present for some years—changes in the respiratory tract may take place, which should be assessed by your doctor. He may decide that such changes need additional treatment.

While the cause of bronchial asthma is allergic, factors other than contact with an allergen are involved in bringing on an attack. Some of these are exposure to irritating fumes or thick smog and changes in temperature or in the humidity in the air. And particularly, emotional stress can precipitate an attack or spell.

The reason that, unlike in hay fever, antihistamines do not bring relief is that the spasm in bronchial asthma is not necessarily induced by histamine. Other substances to which the individual is intolerant may be the cause. Since there is no histamine to block or to antagonize, the antihistamines lie unemployed and their histamine-blocking skill is unused.

What is desperately needed in an attack of bronchial asthma is to open the air passages—not in the nose as in hay fever, but in the respiratory apparatus in the chest, in the small bronchial tubes. There is a double need: to dilate the tubes and to cough up sputum or phlegm. Relief follows almost immediately.

Perhaps the best way to control bronchial asthma is to prevent it—often easier said than done. One way is to dispose of the offending allergen. It can be the house dog or cat, birds, feathers, or material that is part of upholstery or other furniture. Elimination of smoking (*not* reduction but elimination) is helpful. Promoting a good state of health is as important; that is a many-sided task—also more easily said than done.

INGREDIENTS

With the need in bronchial asthma to dilate bronchial tubes, the medicines used in its relief and control are naturally directed to that end.

The medications are of two kinds: tablets and sprays. Sprays are for the immediate need to overcome the paroxysm by oral inhalation. They usually work almost instantly.

Theophylline is a standard ingredient in the tablet or capsule preparations for the control or relief of bronchial asthma—and rightly so. It relaxes muscles in the walls of the bronchial tubes and can be used to help prevent an attack.

Ephedrine dilates the bronchial tubes (though it constricts capillaries in the nostrils). Usually, theophylline and ephedrine are combined in one tablet—a good combination.

Some tablets contain antihistamines, as methapyrilene or thenyldiamine. Although antihistamines are usually not useful in the paroxysm of bronchial asthma, they produce drowsiness, hence they relax.

Occasionally products contain phenobarbital, only 1/8 grain (8 mg.). The dose is so small because products containing more than that amount per tablet cannot be sold over-the-counter without prescription. There is another and better reason for a small dose of phenobarbital: in large doses it depresses respiration. This depressing effect is not pronounced in the customary doses when used as a sedative. People with bronchial asthma cannot tolerate drugs that depress respiration; they need respiratory stimulation not depression.

Another ingredient is glyceryl guaiacolate. This is an expectorant (see *Expectorants and Cough Suppressants*) reducing the viscosity of mucus, helping to expel it.

Do not take a medication that contains belladonna. Belladonna is a desirable ingredient in a preparation for hay fever, because it reduces nasal secretion—fine in runny nose. But in bronchial asthma it is highly undesirable just because it reduces secretions, making mucus thicker and harder to expel by coughing. The objective is to increase secretion with an expectorant such as glyceryl guaiacolate, ammonium chloride, or terpin hydrate to make mucus thinner.

The reason belladonna is used at times as an ingredient in bronchial asthma preparations is that it also dilates bronchial tubes. But the drying side effect cancels out the good it may do. In fact, even in coughs associated with the common cold, belladonna is not a desirable ingredient in the presence of sputum or phlegm which should be brought up.

Asthma cigarettes (now sold only on prescription) which contained belladonna had the same fault. Absorption by inhalation is in fact much more rapid than taking medication by the oral route. (This does not apply to all drugs.)

Other products available over-the-counter without prescription are sprays, for oral inhalation for the rapid control of bronchial asthma attacks. They owe their effect to epinephrine

(Adrenalin). This is not ephedrine. Each spray contains a premeasured amount and must be used cautiously, with respect to frequency and quantity. The package circulars give considerable detail and should be read closely before using these sprays. As previously mentioned, though available over-the-counter they should not be used unless a physician has so advised, because some of the unwanted effects of the epinephrine sprays can be dangerous.

If Your Need Is for a Product Against Bronchial Asthma:

Look for Products Containing the Following Ingredients:

For Oral Use
- Theophylline
- Methapyrilene
- Ephedrine
- Glyceryl guaiacolate

For Inhalation (with caution)
- Epinephrine

NAMES OF PRODUCTS

CAPSULES OR TABLETS AGAINST BRONCHIAL ASTHMA

Asthmanefrin Capsules (Thayer)—Contains theophylline, pseudoephedrine, methapyrilene hydrochloride 15 mg., and glyceryl guaiacolate.

Bronitin Tablets (Whitehall)—Contains theophylline, ephedrine hydrochloride, methapyrilene hydrochloride 16 mg., and glyceryl guaiacolate.

Bronkaid Tablets (Sterling)—Contains ephedrine sulfate, theophylline, thenyldiamine hydrochloride, and glyceryl guaiacolate.

Bronkotabs Tablets (Breon)—Contains ephedrine sulfate 24 mg., glyceryl guaiacolate 100 mg., theophylline 100 mg., phenobarbital 8 mg., and thenyldiamine hydrochloride 10 mg.

Primatene Tablets (Whitehall)—Contains theophylline, ephedrine hydrochloride, and phenobarbital 1/8 gr. (8 mg.).

Tedral Tablets (Warner-Chilcott)—Contains theophylline 130 mg., ephedrine hydrochloride 24 mg., and phenobarbital 8 mg.

INHALANT SPRAYS AGAINST BRONCHIAL ASTHMA FOR ORAL INHALATION

Asthmanephrin Aerosol Mist (Thayer)—Contains *racemic** epinephrine hydrochloride 8.3 mg./1 cc.;† each spray or puff delivers approximately 0.3 mg. racemic epinephrine.

Bronkaid Aerosol Mist (Sterling)—Contains epinephrine hydrochloride 5.5 mg./1 cc.; each spray or puff delivers approximately 0.2 mg. epinephrine.

Primatene Aerosol Mist (Whitehall)—Contains epinephrine 5.5 mg./1 cc.; each spray or puff delivers approximately 0.2 mg. epinephrine.

HAY FEVER

DEFINITION

Hay fever is an allergic condition usually occurring in summer and fall, consistent with the seasonal presence of pollen in the air. It is characterized by much sneezing, itching and tearing eyes and either running or congested nostrils.

CAUSE

Allergic predisposition and sensitivity (*hyper*sensitivity) to the offending pollen or other allergic stimulant.

DISCUSSION AND CAUTIONS

Allergy is a systemic disease in that it can manifest itself in different organs of the body. Our immediate concern in this section is hay fever. Therein, the allergy manifests itself in discomfort in the nose and eyes.

* Racemic epinephrine is weaker than the normal (*l*) form which is regular or standard epinephrine. Hence, while the 8.3 mg. of racemic is not stronger than the 5.5 mg. of regular epinephrine it is about the same strength or effectiveness as the regular epinephrine (more precisely identified as the *l* form). Epinephrine is better known under its trademarked name of Adrenalin.

† If the strength of such inhalant solutions is given in terms of percentage, please note: 5.5 mg. per 1 cc. is equivalent to 0.5% (1 cc. is the same as 1 ml.; the latter is currently preferred usage).

Allergy is a heightened or increased sensitivity (*hyper*sensitivity). The allergic person responds disproportionately, strongly, to a stimulus. The method of reducing this sensitivity is by desensitization, which means giving the minutest doses of the substance to which a person is sensitive, then gradually increasing the doses by minute increments. Desensitization, a long process, often reduces sensitivity. But the pollen or other substance to which the individual is oversensitive must first be found in order to be able to start the desensitization process.

Aside from desensitization, the treatment of hay fever is directed merely to relief of the symptoms—i.e., to allay the discomfort in the eyes and nose. There is no simple cure for hay fever. Desensitization (which is really *hypo*sensitization, making a person less sensitive) does not cure either. It only alleviates symptoms which usually return when hyposensitization is stopped. Physicians usually advocate hyposensitization if the allergic person cannot be made comfortable by antihistamines.

The relief of symptoms usually follows an antihistamine taken orally and a decongestant sprayed into the nose. Antihistamines work by antagonizing or blocking histamine. The latter is liberated as a result of the allergic reaction. Antihistamines work well in the allergic reaction as manifested in seasonal hay fever (there are also other manifestations of allergy).

The decongestants, as ephedrine, do not block antihistamines but they work by constricting the swollen mucous membrane of the nostrils, as in colds (see *The Common Cold*). They are used largely in the form of nasal spray. Both a decongestant nasally and an antihistamine orally can be used at the same time.

INGREDIENTS

The antihistamines used orally are usually methapyrilene fumarate, pheniramine maleate, chlorpheniramine maleate, or pyrilamine maleate.

The decongestants used in the nasal sprays are much the

same as those used for the relief of cold symptoms: phenylephrine hydrochloride (Neo-Synephrine), naphazoline (Privine), and phenylpropanolamine hydrochloride (Propadrine). They constrict the vessels in the nostrils, clearing passage for air in breathing.

Belladonna or atropine is at times used as a component in tablets taken to relieve hay fever symptoms—coryza or rhinitis tablets are examples. Here, also, a side effect is taken advantage of: belladonna dries secretions, reducing nasal discharge.

Some products contain aspirin, which is useful only if there is an accompanying headache. It does not do anything for hay fever symptoms. A few products contain acetanilid: *Avoid them.* Acetanilid has been taken out of most over-the-counter products, as it may produce methemoglobinemia, a condition in which the hemoglobin cannot carry oxygen.

There is very little difference among the antihistamines and, in fact, among the decongestants in the over-the-counter products available without prescription. One product may work better in a given individual, another product in a different individual. There is no predictability, since these are individual variations. (See also *The Common Cold* for the cautions regarding decongestants.)

If Your Need Is for a Product Against Hay Fever:

Look for Products Containing the Following Ingredients:

Methapyrilene
Pheniramine
Chlorpheniramine
Pyrilamine

(For decongestants in clearing nasal passages, see table on pages 47–48.)

NAMES OF PRODUCTS

CAPSULES OR TABLETS FOR HAY FEVER

Note: Please refer to decongestants under *The Common Cold* (pages 50–51); all of these of course, contain a decongestant, and most of them also contain an antihistamine. They are equally suitable in hay fever. The products listed below are labeled for use in hay fever; some contain only antihistamines.

Allerest Tablets (Pennwalt) —Contains phenylpropanolamine hydrochloride 25 mg., chlorpheniramine maleate 1 mg., and methapyrilene fumarate 5 mg.

Inhiston (Pharmaco) —Contains pheniramine maleate.

Kriptin (Whitehall) —Contains pyrilamine maleate.

NASAL DECONGESTANT SPRAYS

Note: Please refer to nasal decongestant sprays under *The Common Cold* (pages 51–52), all of which contain a decongestant and most of which contain decongestant and antihistamine. They are equally suitable for use in hay fever.

SKIN

The skin is subject to many problems and dysfunctions. Many are amenable to self-treatment by drugs available over-the-counter. The obvious ones include itching, baby skin irritations, sunburn, minor burns, poison ivy, psoriasis, age spots, athlete's foot, dandruff, and acne.

But there are over-the-counter products obtainable without prescription which are offered for the self-treatment of other skin conditions. One of them is eczema. We have intentionally omitted any discussion of eczema. The reason is not necessarily based on safety; by and large the product will probably not be harmful and, in fact, may even relieve some itches in eczema. But eczema is a complex condition. First, there are various types of eczema. Second, there are various causes for it—for example, allergy is the cause of one type. You have to know what you are dealing with in order to maximize usefulness. For that reason see your physician if you have eczema. This applies to children as well as adults.

There is another reason why we do not consider a number of other skin conditions. That reason is based on the fact that skin conditions can also be a manifestation of an internal condition. See *The Skin as Signal of Disease* (page 227).

ITCH

DEFINITION

An itch is an unpleasant sensation on the skin which generates a desire to scratch. And scratching often causes a more intense, painful sensation.

CAUSE

An itch may be due to a variety of causes, each of which stimulates the nerve endings in the skin. This stimulation expresses itself in an itch. It can be the result of irritation from clothes, as wool or infections of the skin. It may be produced by drugs, either taken internally or applied on the skin. It may accompany other diseases, as Hodgkin's disease, jaundice, or kidney disease. Itch can also be caused by dryness of the skin due to low humidity, so-called winter itch. Other causes may be psychological; people with psychological problems will sometimes have physical manifestations of their anxieties, and one of them is frequently an itch.

DISCUSSION AND CAUTIONS

Why it is more respectable to have a pain than an itch is not clear. Scratching in the presence of others to alleviate an itch labels one a boor. Holding a painful site or rubbing it does not carry social disapproval. Perhaps the reason lies in the cultural stereotype we have inherited. Yet itching and pain carry many similarities.

An itch may be perceived anywhere in the body—even on hard skin, except on a callus. At times an itch is such a generalized feeling that while it is felt on a broad area of the body, such as the back or the face, the spot cannot easily be located.

Only epidermis can itch. An area denuded of skin does not itch; one cannot produce an itch on a place that has been excoriated. When the healing process begins, an itch sensation often accompanies it.

There is a considerable psychological component in itching. For example, a discussion about itching occasionally creates the sensation of an itch, and people attempt to scratch without being aware of doing so. It is believed that people susceptible to itching are emotionally more volatile than those who are not. Many chronic skin conditions are believed to have a substantial psychological underlay.

An itch often improves when attention is focused on an activity outside of ourselves, which reveals the psychological underlay of itching. Yet, certain conditions of the skin are more susceptible to itching, as dry skin or aging skin. And scratching is not necessarily a relief, because the irritation that can be caused by scratching can make skin raw, and this can make the itch worse.

A particular type of itch is *pruritus ani,* which means itching of the anus. This is often associated with hemorrhoids (page 96), but there may be other reasons for this particular itch, as emotional upset, worms, the result of antibiotic therapy, allergy, or a fungal infection.

The itch of athlete's foot, while it is often intense, can be ameliorated with the athlete's foot remedies available (see later discussion).

The skin is subject to various types of infection, another possible cause of itch. Infections can be caused by bacteria, viruses, fungi, or parasites.

Among the common bacterial infections are boils, impetigo, and other skin diseases characterized by pustules. The fungal infections include athlete's foot and ringworm. In the viral infections, such as in the cold sore or fever sore (herpes simplex) or shingles (herpes zoster), there is associated itching. Infections with parasites also can occur, as in scabies, which is an infection with the skin mite.

INGREDIENTS

Except for local anesthetics, which usually obtund itching, relief of itching is not necessarily predictable. For some an application of cold, for others heat, relieves itching. For that reason menthol, which cools on application, is usually an ingredient in preparations for the relief of an itch. But a liniment, especially one that confers a sensation of warmth (see under *Muscle Pain,* page 122), may also relieve an itch, though paradoxically liniments irritate the skin. Pure glycerine, when lightly rubbed on the skin, also gives a feeling of warmth. It is not as irritating as a liniment, and upon repeated application it may dry the skin, but dilutions with water will prevent the drying. However, dilutions are not warming. As a rule, liquid applications applied to the skin tend to cool, owing to their aqueous, alcoholic, or menthol content. On the other hand, ointments tend to heat or warm, unless they have a relatively high proportion of menthol or camphor.

Starch or oatmeal baths are commonly used to relieve itching; usually they make the itch milder, but do not necessarily dissipate it.

Alcohol, 15% to 50%, usually found in skin preparations, cools and may mitigate an itch.

Antihistamines, as methapyrilene hydrochloride or chlorpheniramine maleate, often reduce an itch if it is an allergic reaction. But at times antihistamines can paradoxically increase an itch, by sensitizing skin. Phenol (carbolic acid), in about a 2% solution, often does reduce an itch because it mildly anesthetizes the nerve endings. Local anesthetics, as benzocaine or dibucaine (Nupercaine), are usually effective in temporarily relieving an itch. But it should be borne in mind that local anesthetics can sensitize, irritate, and make matters worse.

Many products for the skin which have substantially the same formula are often offered for different conditions, such as acne, itching, dandruff, and for healing. There may be several reasons for this: (1) the art of mitigating skin discomforts is empirical—a product may have been found useful on long experience; (2) tradition; (3) a variety of skin conditions are treated by the same remedy, as an antiseptic. For example, an antiseptic that conceivably promotes healing by preventing infection or reinfection is also useful as an ingredient in a detergent preparation for the removal of dandruff.

Even products suitable for different uses and made by the same manufacturer may differ only slightly. For example, Medicone Derma Ointment contains exactly the same several ingredients as the Medicone Rectal Unguent, with the following exception: the Derma Ointment contains ichthammol, a sulfur containing material, whereas the Rectal Unguent contains balsam Peru. Both ingredients are quite similar, as auxiliaries, in their mildly antiseptic and stimulating effect.

It is not to be understood that itching is a hopeless condition. It can be ameliorated. It should merely be borne in mind that frequently one cannot foretell what product will ameliorate an itch without at times producing a skin reaction that can make an itch worse.

The base of an ointment is the vehicle in which the so-called active ingredients are incorporated. The base is most frequently composed of a mixture of petrolatum (such as Vaseline), water, stearic acid, cetyl alcohol, lanolin or lanolin extractives, with water. These bases are emollient or softening, and may be useful for a mild itch without the usual active ingredients, such as zinc oxide, phenol, benzocaine, menthol, and camphor.

If Your Need Is for a Product Against Itching:

Look for Products Containing the Following Ingredients:

- Alcohol
- Benzocaine
- Dibucaine

NAMES OF PRODUCTS

Nupercainal Ointment (Madison/Ciba)—Contains dibucaine hydrochloride 1%. (Also available as Nupercainal Pain Relief Lotion containing 0.5% dibucaine, and Spray containing 0.25% dibucaine.)

Zemo Liquid (Plough)—Contains phenol, sodium salicylate, menthol, methyl salicylate, borax, thymol, eucalyptol, and alcohol 35%. Offered as an antiseptic against "itching."

Zemo Extra Strong Liquid (Plough)—The ingredients, as well as conditions for which it is offered, are the same as above, except that this "extra strong" solution contains 40% alcohol against the 35% of the regular strength. Presumably, the small extra addition of alcohol is used to dissolve slightly more of the alcohol-soluble ingredients, though this is not conclusive, as the amounts of ingredients are not given on the label.

Calamatum Spray (Blair)—Contains benzocaine 0.5%, calamine, zinc oxide, menthol, camphor, and isopropyl alcohol 9.4%.

BABY SKIN PROBLEMS

DEFINITION

The most prominent problems to which baby skin is subject are diaper rash, prickly heat, and heat rash. These skin irritations usually are accompanied by itching or a sense of burning.

CAUSE

Diaper rash is a skin irritation that arises from decomposition of the urine in contact with skin by a wet diaper. Prickly heat or heat rash is a rash often accompanied by itching or pinhead-size bumps on the skin, due to blocked sweat ducts.

DISCUSSION AND CAUTIONS

When urine is exposed to the air, especially when in a warm environment, it decomposes, one of the products being ammonia. These are exactly the conditions that occur when a wet diaper remains long in contact with a baby's warm skin. Skin irritation, accompanied by itching and burning, can be extremely uncomfortable. Prickly heat, on the other hand, can occur in adults as well as in infants. In infants it is likely to occur especially in warm weather when perspiration is increased. Comparatively minor conditions can produce it.

Both diaper rash and prickly heat, especially when mild, are remedied without too much effort; but the difficulty resides when the diaper is too long in contact with skin and frequently wetted anew.

The best treatment for both diaper rash and prickly heat is prevention. The use of powder as an absorbent of perspiration is also a preventive measure. Skin oil is an alternate preventative: while it does not absorb perspiration, it does tend to keep the skin dry.

INGREDIENTS

Frequently a bland ointment, containing petrolatum (Vaseline) with a small amount of lanolin, is sufficient to allay irritation of prickly heat. However, a bland ointment containing vitamins A and D may be preferable. Often ointments and powders are effective because of the mechanical barrier they present to such irritation as chafing.

The materials used in ameliorating baby skin irritations can be conveniently divided into four groups: (a) antiseptics and germicides, (b) mechanical agents such as powders, (c) lubricants such as mineral oil, and (d) ointments. They serve a variety of purposes in either prevention or self-treatment or both.

Among detergents to make cleansing more efficient is sodium octylphenoxyethoxyethyl ether sulfonate, also known in some brands as Entsufon. (See also skin cleansers under *Acne,* pages 216–17.)

Among the antiseptics are hexachlorophene, methyl benzethonium chloride, benzalkonium chloride, and certain phenolic antiseptics as chloroxylenol or phenol, or occasionally 8-hydroxyquinoline. They are used in minute amounts to reduce the likelihood of diaper rash and are rarely irritating. However, if a combination of two or more antiseptics is used there is an increased probability of irritation or, particularly, sensitization. The reason given for using two or more antiseptic ingredients instead of one is that the probability of irritation is reduced because less of each is used. The hypothesis is attractive and perhaps logical. But the possibility of sensitization is nonetheless increased.

Powders act as mechanical agents (though some of them may have an additional activity independent of their mechanical effect, such as an antiseptic effect). For example, in chafing, a powder acts as a mechanical interface coating the irritated skin, with a residual surface of powder between apposing skin sites.

The effect of talcum is mechanical, hence protective. It does not absorb moisture as well as cornstarch, but the small amount of moisture it does take up, and the mechanical coating it offers, make it a useful application to baby skin surfaces.

Boric acid used in ointments and in powders is theoretically an antiseptic, though reliance cannot be placed on that effect in the proportion used. But it is a fine mechanical aid since it is slippery.

Zinc oxide is used in both ointments and powders. It is a good addition since it is slightly antiseptic and drying. Magnesium carbonate is not antiseptic but is drying.

Cornstarch absorbs moisture, and is a good mechanical aid. It is a better absorbent than talcum. For chafing it is therefore superior to talcum. But cornstarch, due to its greater absorbing ability, is more likely to cake than talcum.

Zinc stearate is an outstandingly good baby powder. It is water-repellent and thus prevents contact between skin and urine, precluding diaper rash. It is not currently popular, as other powders have caught the public fancy. As with books, the best-sellers are not necessarily the most enduring books. However good it is for the stated purpose, it should be used with caution because although it does not hurt the baby on application, it can hurt the mother and the child—*if they inhale it.* It is easy enough to inhale it if dusted generously making a cloud. But careful dusting on a diaper or gentle application on skin prevents a cloud of powder, and eliminates the danger. This applies to the use of any dusting powder.

Magnesium stearate is water-repellent and a small amount is used in powders to ward off water.

Alum is an astringent and is infrequently used in body powders. Salicylic acid is antiseptic and is probably useful in prickly heat, but it tends to make skin softer and in larger amounts can soften the epidermis and be distinctly irritating. Bismuth subcarbonate or subnitrate is a protective and mechanical aid. However, in the small amounts that bismuth salts are used in these powders, the principal effect is that produced by the basic ingredient, talc or cornstarch.

Mineral oil is the principal oil used in baby preparations. It is a good lubricant, does not turn rancid, and is also protective for mechanical reasons. Lanolin is an ingredient used in small proportion in baby oils and does not really add substantially to the total effect of a baby oil. Oils are generally useful to repel water.

The term *lanolin cholesterols* refers to an extract of lanolin, with the same skin-softening effect of lanolin. Petrolatum, for which Vaseline is a trade name, is merely solid mineral oil, as mineral oil is a liquid fraction of petrolatum. Paraffin is a harder petrolatum, and paraffin oil is the same as mineral oil. Ceresin is a wax.

A good baby powder principally contains talcum, with or without small amounts of cornstarch. A good baby oil principally contains mineral oil and an antiseptic, particularly if it is also intended to treat diaper rash. Baby ointments, which are essentially solid forms of the oils, are offered for a variety of skin conditions such as chafing, prickly heat, chapping, diaper rash, or minor skin irritations. Ointments often contain additional ingredients such as vitamins A and D and, at times, pantothenol, which aid healing.

If Your Need Is for a Product Against Diaper Rash:

Look for Products Containing the Following Ingredients:

- Petrolatum
- Vitamins A and D
- Talcum

Cornstarch
Zinc stearate
Mineral Oil
Hexachlorophene
Methylbenzethonium chloride
Benzethonium chloride
Benzalkonium chloride
8-Hydroxyquinoline

NAMES OF PRODUCTS

PRODUCTS FOR BABY SKIN IRRITATIONS

A and D Cream (White) —Contains vitamins A and D, hexachlorophene, in a base of lanolin.

Ammens Medicated Powder (Bristol-Myers) —Contains 8-hydroxyquinoline and talc. Offered for diaper rash.

Balmex Baby Powder (Macsil) —Contains balsam Peru, vitamins A and D, zinc oxide, bismuth subnitrate; base contains silicone. Also available in lotion or ointment.

Comfortine Medicated Ointment (Rorer) —Contains calamine, zinc oxide, and boric acid in lanolin base.

Cradol (Sterling) —Contains hexachlorophene in emulsified petrolatum base.

Desitin Baby Powder (Pfizer) —Contains hexachlorophene, chloroxylenol, and talcum.

Desitin Medicated Baby Oil (Pfizer) —Contains mineral oil, hexachlorophene, and chloroxylenol.

Desitin Ointment (Pfizer) —Contains cod liver oil (vitamins A and D), zinc oxide, lanolin, petrolatum, and talcum.

Diaparene Antibacterial Baby Lotion (Sterling) —Contains methylbenzethonium chloride in emulsified base.

Diaparene Baby Powder (Sterling) —Contains methylbenzethonium chloride, cornstarch, and magnesium carbonate.

Diaparene Ointment (Sterling) —Contains methylbenzethonium chloride, petrolatum, and glycerine.

Johnson's Baby Cream (Johnson & Johnson) —Contains mineral oil, paraffin, lanolin, and white beeswax ceresin.

Johnson's Baby Lotion (Johnson & Johnson)—Contains hexachlorophene in lanolin-containing lotion.

Johnson's Baby Oil (Johnson & Johnson)—Contains mineral oil and lanolin.

Johnson's Baby Powder (Johnson & Johnson)—Contains talcum.

Johnson's Medicated Powder (Johnson & Johnson)—Contains calcium silicate, talc, and hexachlorophene.

Maroc Baby Powder (Maroc)—Contains benzalkonium chloride, hexachlorophene, zinc silicofluoride, magnesium carbonate, and kaolin.

Medicated Comfort Powder (Parke, Davis)—Contains talc, cornstarch, alum, magnesium carbonate, salicylic acid, phenol, and hexachlorophene.

Mennen Baby Magic Bath (Mennen)—Contains hexachlorophene.

Mennen Baby Magic Conditioning Oil (Mennen)—Contains mineral oil and lanolin.

Mennen Baby Magic Lotion (Mennen)—Contains lanolin and benzalkonium chloride.

Mennen Baby Magic Powder (Mennen)—Contains methylbenzethonium chloride and talc.

Mexsana Medicated Powder (Plough)—Contains cornstarch, hexachlorophene, kaolin, zinc oxide, oil of eucalyptus, and camphor.

Petroleum Jelly (Various Manufacturers)—(Vaseline.)

pHisoHex (Winthrop)—Contains hexachlorophene and Entsufon.

Tashan Skin Cream (Sauter/Hoffmann-LaRoche)—Contains vitamins A and D, pantothenol, and vitamin E.

Tod'l Antibacterial Lotion (Sterling)—Contains Entsufon, lanolin cholesterols, petrolatum, and hexachlorophene.

Z.B.T. Baby Powder (Sterling)—Contains talc, mineral oil, and magnesium stearate.

BURNS

DEFINITION

A burn is skin damage resulting from exposure to any strong source of heat, particularly hot water or steam, fire, electricity, certain chemicals, or x-ray.

CAUSE

Exposure to too much heat from whatever source produces a burn. Burns can also occur through friction, as sliding down a rope or a long slide without adequate protective clothing.

DISCUSSION AND CAUTIONS

Burns can be life-threatening when they are over an extensive part of the body or burn tissues more deeply than the skin. The reason for their seriousness is not due to the intensive pain—that can be handled—but due to the loss of water and salts and impending shock. Extensive or deep burns can be especially serious to diabetics, the aged, or when the burned person has heart or kidney disease. This is particularly true when there is inhalation of hot gases, as in a fire.

One of the ways by which burns are classified is by degree: in a first-degree burn there are redness and pain, even swelling or edema but no blistering; in a second-degree burn there is blistering in addition. In a third-degree burn there is intense pain, with destruction of the skin and often damage to deeper tissue which does not necessarily show blisters.

The only type of burn that can be self-treated is the first-degree burn and, perhaps, when there is a blister (second-degree) over a small area.

Various remedies can be used in the casual burn received in the kitchen, workshop, or elsewhere in the house. Make no mistake about it: the casual burn may be quite painful. Keeping a burned hand under cold water, or applying ice cubes, sterile petrolatum, or even butter will be helpful until a more satisfactory remedy can be obtained.

When a book of matches flares up while being held it can produce a blistered, severe and painful burn. It has the marks of a powder burn, and may require an antitetanus injection after the immediate measures are taken to relieve the pain.

Burns easily become infected, as the microorganisms normally present on skin or in nostrils can cause an infection in the presence of dead or damaged skin. A burn, especially if blistered, should therefore be bandaged or otherwise covered to prevent infection. Any medication that is used should be sterile. For example, the contents of a jar of "burn ointment" should not be used—fingers put in on a previous occasion have probably introduced bacteria.

Thus, the objective in safe self-treatment of burns is reduction of pain, keeping the burned site from infection, and allowing the skin to heal naturally.

If a person who has suffered a burn, even a small one, develops fever or unusual fatigue a few days after a burn—or even earlier—he may be developing an infection. In that case it is imperative to see a physician.

INGREDIENTS

There are numerous ingredients in burn remedies. Most of these ingredients are superfluous. What is basically needed is an antiseptic and a local anesthetic. Many preparations offered for burns also carry claims for use for other conditions such as cuts, scrapes, minor insect bites, poison ivy. They are not therefore necessarily better for burns. It is wiser not to complicate self-treatment of burns by using products that contain zinc oxide or aluminum hydroxide. While they are not necessarily harmful, they do not contribute to what is needed in burn treatment, which is, specifically, reducing pain and preventing infection.

Among antiseptics are benzalkonium chloride, hexachlorophene, methylbenzethonium chloride, isooctylphenoxypolyethanol (one of the Triton products, which are surface-active and antiseptic), and orthophenyl phenol (Dowicide 1).

Some otherwise reliable antiseptics are less effective for burns because to be safe they must be used in quantities smaller than optimum. This is especially true in combination with the other ingredients in the preparations. Examples of these are carbolic acid and other phenols. Some have greater antiseptic power than phenol, and in effect they can be grouped together: parachlorometaxylenol, hexylated metacresol, and chlorothymol. Two of them with mercury, mercurimetacresol and orthochloromercuriphenol, are probably better due to the mercury content.

Local anesthetics include lidocaine (Xylocaine), benzocaine, dibucaine (Nupercaine), butacaine (Butesin), and diperodon (Diothane). All local anesthetics may possibly sensitize, but when pain relief is necessary, that chance may be wise to take.

Aerosols are a convenient form of application. Most of them contain alcohol for solubilizing the ingredients. Bear in mind, however, that some will sting momentarily due to the alcohol content.

If Your Need Is for a Product Against Burns:

Look for Products Containing the Following Ingredients:

- Butesin picrate
- Benzocaine
- Dibucaine
- Benzalkonium chloride
- Hexachlorophene
- Orthophenylphenol

NAMES OF PRODUCTS

AGAINST BURNS

Bactine Aerosol (Miles)—Contains lidocaine, isopropyl alcohol, methylbenzethonium chloride, isooctylphenoxypolyethanol, and chlorothymol.

Bactine Antiseptic Liquid (Miles)—Contains methylbenzethonium chloride, chlorothymol, isooctylphenoxypolyethanol, and alcohol 13%.

Butesin Picrate Ointment (Abbott)—Contains 1% butesin picrate.

Medi-Quik First Aid Spray (Sterling)—Contains lidocaine, benzalkonium chloride, hexachlorophene, and isopropyl alcohol (12%).

Nupercainal Pain Relief Lotion (Madison)—Contains 0.5% dibucaine.

Nupercainal Pain Relief Spray (Madison)—Contains 0.25% dibucaine and alcohol 46%.

Solarcaine Cream (Plough)—Contains benzocaine, orthophenylphenol, hexachlorophene, camphor, and menthol.

Solarcaine Spray (Aerosol) (Plough)—Contains benzocaine, orthophenylphenol, hexachlorophene, and isopropyl alcohol 7%.

Un-Burn Aerosol (Leeming/Pacquin)—Contains benzocaine, hexachlorophene, chloroxylenol, and menthol.

Un-Burn Cream (Leeming/Pacquin)—Contains benzocaine, hexachlorophene, orthophenylphenol, and menthol.

Unguentine Aerosol (Norwich)—Contains benzocaine, benzalkonium chloride, parachlorometaxylenol, phenol, oil of thyme, menthol, oil of eucalyptol, and alcohol 7%.

Unguentine First Aid Aerofilm (Norwich)—Contains benzalkonium chloride, orthochloromercuriphenol 0.006%, parachlorometaxylenol, diperodon, phenol, oil thyme, menthol, oil eucalyptus, eugenol, and alcohol 7%.

Unguentine Ointment (Norwich)—Contains phenol 1%, parahydroxymercurimetacresol, zinc oxide, aluminum hydrate, zinc carbonate, zinc acetate, eucalyptus oil, and thyme oil.

Unguentine Plus (Norwich)—Contains lidocaine hydrochloride, *p*-chlorometaxylenol, aluminum hydrate, zinc carbonate, zinc acetate, zinc oxide, phenol, oil eucalyptus, oil thyme, menthol, and eugenol in cream base.

SUNBURN

DEFINITION

Sunburn is a discomfort that follows exposure to the sun, or to its indirect rays as reflected from snow or water, and is characterized by reddening, burning, and stinging of the skin. It is a first-degree burn.

CAUSE

Direct exposure to sunlight, indirect exposure to it by reflection of its rays by snow or water even through lightly overcast skies, or by exposure to a sunlamp.

DISCUSSION AND CAUTIONS

There is a comparatively narrow range of the spectrum of sunrays that burn—they are short, i.e., 2,900 to 3,200 angstrom units. Heavy smoke and fog filter out sunlight. But light clouds are deceptive as a sunburn is possible with only lightly overcast skies. Sitting indoors before a closed window with the sun streaming in will not cause sunburn, as window glass filters out the burning rays. (Solaria have windows of a special glass that allows most of the burning rays to pass through.)

Sunburn can be temporarily disabling if it is severe. Swelling of the legs, for example, due to sunburn can prevent moving about; and in fact, general malaise and mild fever may make the sufferer feel too ill to want to move around.

It is true that blonds or people with a light complexion burn more easily; they have less pigment in their skin. Skin pigment filters out the sunrays.

The signs and effect of a sunburn can come on in comparatively few minutes due to photosensitization, which is sensitization to light. It can happen by being in the sunlight after taking certain drugs, such as antibiotics, sulfonamides, sometimes phenobarbital or certain tranquilizers, among other drugs. Drugs that sensitize people when they are exposed to sunlight are called photosensitizing drugs. This does not happen to all people, but some have a systemic make-up that makes them more sensitive to the sun.

The burning rays of the sun—actinic rays—are strongest from about 11:00 A.M. to 4:00 P.M., especially in the summer. They can also threaten during the spring or fall, though less so. The first exposure during the summer should not be longer than 20 minutes, with 5 or 10 minute daily increments to build up a pigment layer, called a tan.

A mild degree of sunburn with only little discomfort is evident by redness. A somewhat greater degree is characterized by swelling, then tenderness of the skin or pain, finally blistering, before the very considerable pain and burning subside. The process of peeling that follows has much less discomfort.

Exposure to the sun occasionally gives rise to nausea, weakness, dizziness, fever, and in extreme cases, heat stroke. Heat stroke is often due to physical activity in hot weather and the consequent loss from the body of salt and water by sweating. Use of water and salt tablets prevents heat stroke. But in the event of heat stroke, do not give medication to a person so disabled. Put him in the shade and sprinkle him with cold water while waiting for the doctor. Do not force him to drink water, as he may not be able to swallow.

Cold water compresses are comforting in sunburn. They should be changed every 5 minutes because after that time they do not cool. Cold compresses reduce the feeling of heat in the skin. Do not use rubbing alcohol which, although cooling, can sting on application. A dilution of 2 tablespoonfuls of rubbing alcohol in a glassful of water, and used as a compress, is cooling and does not sting.

Further exposure to the sun should be avoided until the acute sunburn subsides.

The need in sunburn is similar to that of a heat burn, except that in sunburn an application of a local anesthetic is sufficient. This is more important than the use of an antiseptic.

Protection against sunburn is the wise move. An application of fat or oil does filter some of the burning rays, but it is not as efficient as an ointment or lotion containing a sun-filtering agent.

However, products that claim to contain the most efficient filters are not necessarily safeguards against sunburn. They may well contain efficient filters; but in practice, reliance on these products may be a false security, for after swimming most of the application will be washed off. Similarly, perspiration in the hot sun also reduces the effectiveness of the cover that such an application lends. Sun-filtering products should be frequently reapplied while being exposed to the sun.

Tanning preparations that do not contain a sun filter or sun screen *offer a minimal protection against sunburn.* They are intended to hasten a tan. A sunburn eventually turns into a tan, but more slowly.

INGREDIENTS

For relief from the discomfort of sunburn, any of the preparations listed under *Burns* (pages 183–84) can be used.

Sun filters or sun screens in products that purport to guard against sunburn work by filtering out the sunrays of the burning range, i.e., 2,900–3,200 angstrom units.

The only reason we give the jawbreakers, i.e., the long chemical names, in the following list of sun screens is to enable you to recognize a given ingredient which is often listed by different names. For example, some list the ingredient oxybenzone under its long chemical name—like 2-hydroxy-4-methoxybenzophenone. If the reader is aware of both names he is in a better position to decide if a product with an ingredient name of 12 syllables is really three times as good as one with an ingredient name of 4 syllables. If you read the long chemical name on the label you may often find that different products have the same sun screen or sun filtering agent.

The sun filters are represented by paraaminobenzoic acid (4-aminobenzoic acid), menthyl anthranilate, amylparadimethylaminobenzoate, 2-hydroxy-4-methoxybenzophenone (oxybenzone), 2,2′-dihydroxy-4-methoxybenzophenone (dioxybenzone), 2-hydroxy-4-methoxybenzophenone-5-sulfonic acid (sulisobenzone), digalloyl trioleate, isoamyl-*p*-*N*-dimethylaminobenzoate, 2-ethoxyethyl-*p*-methoxycinnamate, menthyl or homomenthyl salicylate, and triethanolamine salicylate.

Titanium dioxide or zinc oxide, when used in a thick ointment containing 10% to 20% of either ingredient, forms a barrier against the actinic rays of the sun.

Dihydroxyacetone does not protect against sunrays but, when applied to the skin, gradually tans it.

Cocoa butter and coconut oil have no special virtue, except that of fats, which guard against sunburn. The advantage that cocoa butter presents is that it melts at body heat; it is the base from which most rectal suppositories are made.

If Your Need Is for a Product Against Sunburn:

(See table under *Burns,* page 183.)

NAMES OF PRODUCTS

SUNBURN PROTECTIVE PRODUCTS CONTAINING ADDED SUN SCREENS

A-fil Cream (Texas Pharm.) —Contains titanium dioxide and menthyl anthranilate each 5%.

Bain de Soleil (Lanvin) —No ingredients listed.

Bravura Cocoa Sun Lotion (Textron) —Contains 2-ethoxyethyl-*p*-methoxycinnamate.

Bronze Lustre (Revlon) —Contains isoamyl-*p*-*N*-dimethyl aminobenzoate.

Coppertone Baby Tan Lotion (Plough) —Contains isoamyl-*p*-dimethylaminobenzoate and homomenthyl salicylate.

Coppertone Noskote Cream (Plough) —No ingredients listed.

Coppertone Q & T Lotion (Plough) —Contains homomenthyl salicylate and dihydroxyacetone.

Coppertone Suntan Lotion (Plough) —Contains homomenthyl salicylate. (Also available as an oil.)

Indoor/Outdoor Tanning Lotion (Sea & Ski) —Contains isoamyl-*p*-*N*-dimethylaminobenzoate and dihydroxyacetone.

Paraaminobenzoic Acid (Various Manufacturers) —Ointment containing 10% in an ointment or emulsion base.

Sea & Ski Tanning Foam (Sea & Ski) —Contains isoamyl-*p*-*N*-dimethylaminobenzoate.

Skolex (J. B. Williams) —No ingredients listed.

Solbar (Person & Covey) —Contains oxybenzone and dioxybenzone, each 3%.

Sundare (Texas Pharm.) —No ingredients listed.

Sungard (Miles) —Contains 10% sulisobenzone.

Sunswept Cream (Neo A-fil Cream) (Texas Pharm.) Contains digalloyl trioleate 3.5%.

Sure Tan (Bonne Bell) —Contains triethylaminosalicylate.

Tanya Sunburn Preventive (Tanya Hawaii Corp.) —Contains homomenthyl salicylate (in lotion, cream, and spray).

Titanium Dioxide Ointment (Various Manufacturers) —Ointment containing 10% to 20% titanium dioxide. Useful for small areas such as lips. It is too messy to apply and remove over a wide area of the skin.

Weatherproofer (Bonne Bell)—Contains amyl-*p*-dimethylaminobenzoate, allantoin, and hexachlorophene. (A pomade for lips.)

Zinc Oxide Ointment (Various Manufacturers)—Ointment containing 20% zinc oxide. Useful for small areas as lips, too messy to apply and remove over a wide area of the skin.

SKIN TANNING PRODUCTS WITHOUT SUN SCREEN, NO INGREDIENTS LISTED

Almay Deep Tanning Cream (Schieffelin)—Hypoallergenic.

Bronztan Lotion (Shulton)

Coppertan Tanning Butter (Plough)

Sea & Ski Tanning Butter (Sea & Ski)—(Also available in lotion or oil.)

(For preparations to relieve the discomforts of sunburn, see under *Burns* (pages 183–84) or *Itch* (pages 174–75).

POISON IVY

DEFINITION

A skin allergy resulting from contact with the sap of the poison ivy plant (or poison oak or poison sumac), characterized by redness and blisters of the skin, usually swelling, and intense itching.

CAUSE

Contact with the ivy (or oak or sumac) plant or sap.

DISCUSSION AND CAUTIONS

Poison ivy contact is familiar enough, but you should bear in mind that it can lead to infection through scratching. Repeated bouts of poison ivy contact can produce a chronic dermatitis, which becomes quite hard to manage.

First-aid manuals recommend that the poison ivy sap should be neutralized with laundry soap and hot water. That is a wise suggestion. But it works only when used almost immediately after contact. The first time that many people learn of the contact is usually after itching and redness have already set in. Soap and water are useless then. Washing with alcohol is a more effective method of removal after exposure, if used immediately after exposure, before the sap has done damage to the skin.

Injury by poison ivy is self-limiting. It disappears after several days to a week. But of utmost importance is relief, both to obtain comfort and to avoid the need to scratch, which often leads to infection. For that reason, a local anesthetic and an antiseptic to help guard against secondary infection are advisable. (Preparations similar to those listed under *Burns* and *Sunburn* are often suitable.)

INGREDIENTS

Benzocaine, dibucaine (Nupercaine), Cyclomethycaine (Surfacaine), and lidocaine (Xylocaine) are local anesthetics, reducing the pain sensation.

Antihistamines are frequent ingredients in preparations for poison ivy. They include diphenhydramine (Benadryl), tripelennamine (Pyribenzamine), and methapyrilene hydrochloride (Histadyl) and are often helpful.

Zirconium oxide, an insoluble material, is specially used in poison ivy preparations because of the cover it forms; zinc oxide and calamine, which are also insoluble substances, are commonly used.

However, it should be borne in mind that in poison ivy dermatitis the skin is already injured, and as a result the chance for sensitization by local anesthetics and antihistamines is increased. However, one must balance the chance of sensitization that *may* occur, against the itching and burning that are *already* being experienced. It seems to us that the decision as to whether to use some relief-giving preparation is clear: use it to counter the trouble you already have, and take a chance on the superimposed irritation which may or possibly may not occur. It is purely a practical matter, and the decision is much like what your reaction might be to the recommendations given in many first-aid books that prevention, by avoiding contact with poison ivy, is the answer. The question is, what-do-you-do-when-you-already-have-poison-ivy?

There have been differences of opinion on the efficacy of poison ivy preparations and as we go to press an announcement by the FDA proposes to withdraw certain of them from the market.

If Your Need Is for a Product Against Poison Ivy Skin Irritation:

Look for Products Containing the Following Ingredients:

- Benzocaine
- Dibucaine
- Diphenhydramine
- Methapyrilene
- Tripelennamine
- Zinc oxide
- Calamine
- Benzalkonium chloride

NAMES OF PRODUCTS

AGAINST POISON IVY

Antivy Lotion (Madison)—Contains Pyribenzamine (tripelennamine) 2%, zirconium oxide 4%, with methyl and propyl paraben.

Caladryl Lotion (Parke, Davis)—Contains calamine and 1% Benadryl (diphenhydramine), camphor, and 2% alcohol. (Also as cream or spray.)

Calamatum Aerosol (Blair)—Contains zirconium oxide 2%, benzocaine 0.5%, methapyrilene hydrochloride 0.028%, calamine, camphor, and isopropyl alcohol 8.4%.

Calamatum Lotion (Blair)—Contains calamine, zinc oxide, phenol, camphor, benzocaine 3%, and methapyrilene hydrochloride 0.25%.

Calamine Lotion (Various Manufacturers)—Contains calamine, zinc oxide, and phenol.

Caligesic Analgesic Ointment (Quinton/Merck)—Contains calamine 8%, benzocaine 3%, and hexylated metacresol 0.05%.

Medi-Quik First Aid Spray (Sterling)—Contains lidocaine, benzalkonium chloride, hexachlorophene, and isopropyl alcohol 12%.

Nupercainal Pain Relief Lotion (Madison)—Contains 0.5% nupercaine.

Rhulicream (Lederle)—Contains zirconium oxide 1%, benzocaine 1%, menthol, camphor, and alcohol 9%.

Rhulispray (Aerosol) (Lederle)—Contains zirconium oxide 1%, benzocaine, menthol, camphor, calamine, and isopropanol.

Solarcaine Aerosol Spray (Plough)—Contains benzocaine, orthophenyl phenol, hexachlorophene, isopropyl alcohol 7%. (Also in cream and lotion.)

Surfadil Lotion (Lilly)—Contains Histadyl (methapyrilene hydrochloride) 2%, Surfacaine (cyclomethycaine) 0.5%, and titanium dioxide 5%.

Ziradryl Lotion (Parke, Davis)—Contains Benadryl (diphenhydramine) 1%, zirconium oxide 2%, camphor, and alcohol 2%.

PSORIASIS

DEFINITION

The prominent signs of this skin disease are that it is recurrent and chronic, with acute flare-ups and plaques of silvery scales on red areas.

CAUSE: Unknown.

DISCUSSION AND CAUTIONS

Not only the cause of psoriasis is unknown; there is no known cure. Psoriasis improves, recurs, almost disappears but to recur again. While this is a chronic skin disease it has its acute flare-ups, in which redness deepens and more islands of silvery crust become prominent. And itch is prominent.

Psoriasis can occur anywhere on the body, but common sites

are the elbows, knees, nails, and scalp; also the legs and the back.

Since we do not have better therapeutic measures, treatment of psoriasis is directed to two objectives: (a) the amelioration of itch and (b) the elimination of the unsightly psoriatic scales or plaques. In the acute flare-ups the drugs used with the above points in mind are directed to these two objectives. Some of the products are mildly irritating, and a mild irritating quality is desirable to remove the scales. To reduce irritation, application of starch poultices is sometimes found effective. Any measure that reduces inflammation is avidly sought.

After the inflammation has subsided, mildly irritating substances are used and later somewhat more irritating ones. The following equation applies: the more effective the scale-removing material, the more irritating it is likely to be.

But no application for psoriasis improves the condition itself beyond removal of the scales and skin debris, thereby giving the skin an appearance approaching the normal.

INGREDIENTS

The ingredients used in the treatment of psoriasis to remove scales are the following: coal tar, salicylic acid, sulfur, hexachlorophene, allantoin, and occasionally phenol or phenolic substances such as cresol and, more particularly, mercury.

Coal tar is a mild irritant and antiseptic. It is widely used by dermatologists, often successfully, in a number of skin conditions. When used in excess of 5% in a product it can worsen an irritation. For our present purposes, the various coal tar extracts can be considered to have the same effect as coal tar. Preparations using less than 1% coal tar can be used in a mild acute flare-up. Coal tar is a desirable addition to an antipsoriasis product.

Salicylic acid (also benzoic acid) softens and removes skin, hence is used in antipsoriasis preparations to soften and remove scales. That very property makes it irritating, but for practical purposes, in the 1% to 2% proportions used in psoriasis products, its irritating potential is low.

The same comment can be made for sulfur, which is occasionally used as an ingredient. Sulfur differs from salicylic acid or benzoic acid in that it does not soften skin. But sulfur is also antiseptic, and undergoes a chemical change or stimulates a chemical change in the skin, and thereby exerts its effect. The effect of ichthyol, occasionally used as an ingredient in psoriasis preparations, is due largely to sulfur.

Another antiseptic ingredient is hexachlorophene (see also under *Acne* and *Baby Skin Problems*). It is a good addition to antipsoriasis products, as it helps guard against infecting the psoriatic area.

Either phenol or cresol are antiseptic if used in a proportion of 1% to 2% in an aqueous vehicle.

Allantoin is reputed to be a "healing" agent, stimulating the growth of healthy tissue.

Mercury is an effective substance for removal of scales of psoriasis. It should not, however, be used on acutely inflamed skin, but in the care of chronic psoriasis. It does not cure, although the claim is sometimes made. Mercury is available in over-the-counter preparations without prescription for the care of psoriasis as 5% ammoniated mercury ointment or in other forms of mercury.

The forms of the antipsoriasis preparations can be ointments or creams, or liquids which includes lotions. There is little difference in effect among those forms of preparations, except for the advantages the physical form lends. For example, a liquid enters the area among scales more easily; an ointment has the advantage of assuring longer contact between medication and lesion. We often wonder, however, why no surface-active agents—detergents—are incorporated into the liquids used in the treatment of psoriasis.

Another form is an aerosol foam, similar in appearance to shaving cream. We have no idea what advantages that form lends.

An additional type of product for the control of psoriasis by removing the scales, especially on the scalp, is the shampoo. A shampoo form is preferable for washing hair when there are psoriatic lesions on the scalp because it usually contains detergents. But the very nature of use of a shampoo—or medicated soap for that matter—offers only a *limited contact* with the lesion, as it is washed off in a few minutes. There is some antiseptic residual effect if hexachlorophene is one of the ingredients. But the effect of coal tar is largely washed off with the rinsing phase. Some ointments and liquids applied carefully to the scalp assure better contact between lesion and medicine. They can then be washed out hours later.

If Your Need Is for a Product Against Psoriasis:

Look for Products Containing the Following Ingredients:

- Coal tar
- Salicylic acid
- Sulfur
- Ammoniated mercury
- Hexachlorophene

NAMES OF PRODUCTS

Alphosyl Antipsoriatic Lotion (Reed & Carnrick)—Contains crude coal tar extract 5%, allantoin 2%, in greaseless vehicle.

Alphosyl Cream (Reed & Carnrick)—Contains crude coal tar extract 5%, allantoin 2%, in greaseless vehicle.

Alphosyl Shampoo (Tube) (Reed & Carnrick)—Contains special coal tar 5% and hexachlorophene 1%.

Dermoil/Riasol (Shield)—Contains a mercury preparation 0.45%, phenol 0.5%, creosote 0.75% in liquid base.

Mazon Cream (Thayer)—Contains ammoniated mercury 0.08%, benzoic acid, salicylic acid, resorcinol, and tars.

Mazon Medicated Aerosol Foam (Thayer)—Contains ammoniated mercury 0.08%, benzoic acid, salicylic acid, and coal tar extract.

Psorex Cream (Jeffrey Martin Co.)—Contains coal tar 0.5%, allantoin 0.25%, and hexachlorophene 0.25%.

Psorex Shampoo (Jeffrey Martin Co.)—Contains allantoin 0.2%, hexachlorophene 0.1%, and coal tar 0.5%.

Siroil Emulsion (Siroil Labs.)—Contains mercuric oleate (not more than 0.4%), cresol, and mineral oil.

Tar Doak Lotion (Doak)—Coal tar distillate 5% and lactic acid, mineral oil and water.

Tegrin Cream (Block)—Contains allantoin and coal tar extract.
Tegrin Shampoo (Block)—Contains coal tar extract 5%, allantoin 0.2%, and hexachlorophene 1%.

SKIN SPOTS AND BLEACHING CREAMS

DEFINITION

Spots appearing on the skin in people over 40.

CAUSE: Overpigmentation in spots on the skin.

DISCUSSION AND CAUTIONS

Skin pigment (melanin) is what gives the skin its hue or nuance of color. When skin is darkened, as by exposure to the sun, it is due to the fact that the skin stimulates the formation of melanin. (Production of melanin is triggered and influenced by a complex interrelationship of hormonal events that go on in the body. The sun merely mildly stimulates its formation.)

Skin can lose areas of pigmentation, called piebald skin or vitiligo. However, the usual concern, particularly by women, is the small areas of overpigmentation, called age spots. Age spots (also called liver spots, though they have nothing to do with the liver) usually appear on the back of the hand, arms, neck or forehead, ranging in size from that of a pea or smaller to that of a dime. At times they may be generously spread in tiny, frecklelike spots. In fact the tiny areas are freckles, but a different type than the juvenile freckles, though the freckles in the young are also due to too much pigment in certain spots.

These areas of pigmentation begin to appear at about 40 years of age, and tend to increase in size and number with increasing age. They also get darker with time. Usually they are round, but often the disklike roundness has irregular borders.

Women hate those spots. So do men. But women usually try

to get rid of them. Men usually ignore them, or perhaps are unaware of them, as they are unaware of many other skin blemishes.

If these spots are quite dark, with clear margins, there is little that can be done to lighten them. But if the spots are comparatively light, and the margins are not quite clearly demarcated, there are over-the-counter preparations available without prescription which may be used, and sometimes they are useful. But those preparations, called bleaching creams, must not be used over a period of many months for clearing up those spots. They never disappear wholly; at best they just lighten considerably.

At times, the ingredients those preparations contain may cause a mild skin irritation. In that event, stop using the cream that caused it. If you resume, do so with caution if at all. And do not subject any spots that are raised to irritants.

INGREDIENTS

Ammoniated mercury is one ingredient in bleaching creams. It should not be used in strengths greater than 5%. Ammoniated mercury usually does not sensitize and in strengths not greater than 5% rarely irritates. But it should not be used over large areas, only on spot application, because over a large area much mercury may be absorbed. However, ammoniated mercury ointment should not be used in conjunction with iodine or iodine-containing ointments, as the more poisonous mercuric iodide can form.

Some creams contain ammoniated mercury with hexachlorophene. The latter is not particularly necessary, as ammoniated mercury itself is antiseptic; and moreover, a bleaching cream is used to lighten color spots, not to control infection. Hence, hexachlorophene does not make it better.

Another ingredient used is hydroquinone or, at times, monobenzone (monobenzyl ether of hydroquinone). This ingredient is often effective but also irritating. There are no over-the-counter creams, as far as we know, that contain both ammoniated mercury and hydroquinone, and wisely so. The irritation potential would be increased and ammoniated mercury, if reduced to mercury (metallic), can be more readily absorbed and would be toxic.

(People who would be using the spot bleaching creams tend to have dry skin, due to increasing age. They should bear in mind that indoor humidity during the winter, usually low due to heat, tends to dry skin. Age dries skin, so does soap. The use of bath oils, in the bathwater or after bathing, is usually helpful in reducing dryness. Excessive drying can actually produce itching.)

If Your Need Is for a Product Against Skin Spots:

Look for Products Containing the Following Ingredients:
- Ammoniated mercury
- Hexachlorophene
- Hydroquinone

Avoid the Following Ingredients:
- Do not use iodine or any iodine-containing substance when using mercury.

NAMES OF PRODUCTS

BLEACHING CREAMS

Bleach and Glow Cream (Keystone Labs.)—No ingredients listed.

Esoterica Cream, Facial (Mitchum)—Contains ammoniated mercury 1% and hexachlorophene.

Esoterica Cream, Fortified (Mitchum)—Contains ammoniated mercury 3% and hexachlorophene.

Esoterica Cream, Special (Mitchum)—Contains hydroquinone (no proportion given).

Esoterica Cream, Original (Mitchum)—Contains ammoniated mercury 1% and hexachlorophene (same as Esoterica Cream, Facial).

Nadinola Complexion Cream (Chattem)—Contains ammoniated mercury 4%, bismuth subnitrate, and zinc oxide.

Palidia Cream (Mitchum)—No ingredients given.

Stillman's Freckle Cream (Stillman Co.)—Contains ammoniated mercury 4% and bismuth subnitrate.

Ultra Nadinola Cream (Chattem)—Contains hydroquinone (no proportion listed).

FUNGOUS INFECTIONS OF THE SKIN—ATHLETE'S FOOT

DEFINITION

Athlete's foot is a fungous infection of the foot in which there are small blisters and splits of the skin between the toes, with much skin peeling between toes, on soles and heels, accompanied by burning, itching, or stinging. It may also involve the toenails.

CAUSE

Athlete's foot is caused by infection by any of several fungi.

DISCUSSION AND CAUTIONS

Fungi are all around us. They are normally found on the skin, and being dormant create no problems. This is not intended to say that fungi are healthful organisms. But when there is a breakdown or a change in the natural resistance of the body or the skin, a fungous infection can develop. (The organism is the *fungus,* plural *fungi;* the terms *fungous* and *fungal* are adjectives, as in *fungous* infection.)

There are systemic fungous infections, such as blastomycosis, which may be serious. Fungous infections of the skin can be divided into two large classes—i.e., deep fungous infections which undoubtedly should be treated by a physician, and superficial fungous infections, usually athlete's foot, which are often amenable to self-treatment by over-the-counter products available without prescription. Unfortunately, self-treatment sometimes turns into overtreatment.

A skin infection is like a map—which has to be read. Often it is not easy to read the map and determine what skin condition is involved. This is because often several maps are drawn, one on top of the other. A skin condition may be a skin disease upon a skin disease, upon another skin disease.

How does this happen? It takes place when an itching skin disease triggers the irrepressible desire to scratch. Then scratching may infect the original skin condition. Thus the original skin condition may become unrecognizable due to a superimposed infection.

Therefore differentiation of one skin condition from other likely skin conditions becomes important. You should not undertake that, because different conditions may require different treatment.

The skin is a wondrous organ for other reasons. For example, often it is a mirror for internal conditions. Signs on the skin may be actually messengers suggesting what is happening elsewhere in the body. (See *The Skin as Signal of Disease,* pages 227–28.)

A condition that appears to be athlete's foot by its classical signs is not necessarily athlete's foot. Itching, skin peeling, and skin eruptions may have other causes. Is the condition due to scratching and a secondary infection? Is it due to irritation through overgenerous use of medication; or is it due to a drug taken for other purposes? Is it an infection from contact with a household pet? These questions are easier to formulate than the answers.

Athlete's foot (dermatophytosis) is a common condition which is often amenable to self-treatment, if done with care.

Ostensibly, athlete's foot is easily treated and remedied. Practically that is not the case. Athlete's foot may improve, then get worse, and repeat the cycle of improvement and worsening so that it becomes a persistent and troublesome condition.

One of the reasons for its persistence is reinfection. This may occur in the same way and at the same place as the original infection. Reinfection can also take place through shoes worn during the original infection, or often through reinfection from the toenails. Fungi find a resting place under the toenails or at the junction of toenail and skin. When conditions are favorable for reinfection, it can easily occur. Moisture due to perspiration sets up such a condition.

Another complication in self-treatment of athlete's foot is overtreatment. Antifungal preparations are strong skin irritants—necessarily so. Overgenerous use, or application that is too frequent, coupled with poor foot hygiene, can precipitate an inflammation on top of infection. When athlete's foot becomes an inflammation on top of an infection, it has become an acute athlete's foot infection.

In an acutely inflamed condition, the usual athlete's foot preparations should not be used. Instead, sodium bicarbonate solution (2 oz. or approximately 2 heaping tablespoons to 2 quarts of water) or starch foot baths, or cold applications of Burow's solution, and curtailment of walking should reduce the inflammation. After an inflammation subsides, several days or a week of rest should be allowed to pass before the athlete's foot product is used again. Changing to another product may be wise; the other may be better tolerated. And the new product should be used sparingly at first.

In diabetes particularly or in conditions in which circulation to the legs is impeded (peripheral vascular disease), it is particularly important to avoid inflammation or infection. In these conditions athlete's foot should not be self-treated.

No matter what preparation is used, or even if none is used, the following dicta should be observed, both in treatment as well as in prevention:

1. Keep feet dry, particularly the area between toes.
2. Use a foot or dusting powder (talc, starch, etc.) upon drying feet thoroughly after bath or shower.
3. Avoid excessive perspiration by wearing ventilated shoes if possible and preferably avoiding the synthetic leather substitutes which do not "breathe." They are relatively impervious and seal in heat and moisture.

A substance may kill fungi efficiently when subjected to a laboratory test, and it may even be excellent when tested by more than one method. But it does not follow that it will be as effective and predictable as a fungicide when exposed to the variables found under actual conditions, on skin, with its different secretions. For that reason, fungicides, in the context of treatment of athlete's foot, do not necessarily "kill fungi on contact." In this area we can speak only of a substance being somewhat better than another.

INGREDIENTS

There is no magic ingredient among fungicides in alleviating athlete's foot. Any preparation should be used with collateral measures, such as keeping feet dry and avoiding excessive perspiration. The antiseptic ingredients should be, and usually are, both bactericidal and fungicidal.

Undecylenic acid and its salts, such as zinc undecylenate, are fatty acids which are fungicidal. Similarly, other fatty acids—propionic acid or caprylic acid, all of which are found in perspiration—and their zinc or sodium salts also have fungicidal, or at least fungistatic, effects. All of the fatty acids have a low potential for irritation.

Hexachlorophene, an antiseptic widely used, also inhibits fungi and it has the advantage that they do not develop resistance to it.

Thymol and chlorothymol are both bactericidal and fungicidal. However, a doubt exists as to whether they are effective in the small proportions in which they are used, particularly when they are ingredients in an ointment.

Benzoic and salicylic acids, as in Whitfield's ointment, are standard treatment in athlete's foot. The proportion in Whitfield's ointment is benzoic acid 12% and salicylic acid 6%, but the half-strength ointment containing benzoic acid 6% and salicylic acid 3% is preferable, because it is not as irritating. Benzoic acid is a fine fungicide; salicylic is a poor fungicide but it performs an important function as it peels skin. It is necessary to soften and peel away the skin debris in treating athlete's foot. For that reason salicylic acid is a desirable ingredient in any fungicidal preparation.

Iodine, which has been relatively eclipsed by new products, is an excellent fungicidal agent. A 1% alcoholic solution of iodine is available; stronger solutions should not be used unless they are prescribed by a physician. Iodine stains are readily removed by ammonia water.

Sulfur and salicylic acid ointments are also useful fungicides. Usually 1% of each in an ointment form or lotion is not highly irritating.

An ingredient at times found in antifungal preparations is propyl or methyl paraben. These are parahydroxybenzoic acids, used as preservatives, and have a mild antiseptic effect. As an extra ingredient they present no objection. But alone they are not dependable as fungicides.

What fungicide is most preferable for the self-treatment of athlete's foot—ointment, liquid, or powder?

Each form has its advantages and disadvantages, and more than one form can be used. Ointments have the advantage of sticking to the infected zone. However, a fungicidal ingredient is often more effective in a liquid form, especially in an alcoholic solution. An ointment can be more convenient to use at bedtime, and a liquid in the morning (it does not have the "squishy" feeling of ointments). The site can then be dusted with fungicidal powder. Moreover, powders serve a double purpose: they are a vehicle for the fungicidal ingredient and they absorb moisture, which favors keeping a dry zone. A thicker application of ointment is not necessarily more effective than a less generous one: the zone of fungicidal activity is the zone of contact.

Ringworm and jock itch (tinea cruris) are other fungal conditions. Ringworm of the scalp usually occurs in children. In adults, ringworm can occur anywhere on the body. The treatment is the same as for athlete's foot—but is it ringworm? It is often wise to find out by consulting a physician.

Jock itch is confined to the groin—so called because it occurs in the area over which a jock strap is worn (not because it is limited to jockeys; it is not). It is a bacterial or fungal, often a mixed, infection. All conditions that favor a fungal infection are there—moisture from perspiration, heat, friction due to tight or ill-fitting underwear, and a nonventilated area, all adding to the discomfort.

The itching is usually intense. The need to ameliorate it by scratching is usually inhibited; society may allow scratching a face in public, but the groin? Oh no! Hence, the urge to scratch is saved up; if the sufferer survives until he reaches the men's room he scratches until the area is raw.

Soothing applications are usually more necessary than an antifungal agent due to inflammation of the scratched site. Warm baths to which starch is added are comforting. Showers are too fleeting to do any good. Ointments are better not used, since the skin may be macerated from friction, and ointments are heat-retaining. Liquid antifungal agents containing alcohol will sting enough to make one leap heights which would do honor to a ballet dancer. A powder containing an antifungal substance with a low potential of irritation—a salt of undecylenic acid or propionic acid—is more desirable. As in athlete's foot, it is necessary to keep the area dry, to make the environment hostile to fungi. To avoid irritation which triggers itching, woven undershorts should not be worn. Cotton undershorts or preferably nylon undershorts, two sizes too large, are preferable, since they do not cling. They should be changed twice daily. Only cotton pajamas should be used as sleepwear.

Other so-called fungal conditions should not be self-treated. You must know what a condition is before you self-treat.

If Your Need Is for a Fungicide Against Athlete's Foot:

Look for Products Containing the Following Ingredients:

- Benzoic acid
- Salicylic acid
- Hexachlorophene
- Undecylenic acid
- Iodine
- Sulfur
- Tolnaftate

NAMES OF PRODUCTS

ANTIFUNGAL—AGAINST ATHLETE'S FOOT

Absorbine Jr. (Young)—Contains thymol, chloroxylenol, menthol, and acetone.

Calamine Lotion (Various Manufacturers)—Contains calamine and zinc oxide; not fungicidal but at times soothing during the inflammation from overtreatment.

Compound Undecylenic Acid Ointment (Various Manufacturers)—Contains 5% undecylenic acid and 2% zinc undecylenate in an ointment base.

Cruex Spray-On Powder (Pennwalt)—Contains 10% calcium undecylenate and 1% hexachlorophene in talc base (for jock itch).

Desenex Ointment (Pharmacraft)—Contains undecylenic acid 5% and zinc undecylenate 20%.

Desenex Powder (Pharmacraft)—Contains undecylenic acid 2% and zinc undecylenate 20%.

Desenex Solution (Pharmacraft)—Contains undecylenic acid 10%.

Iodine Tincture—Half Strength (Various Manufacturers)—Contains 1% iodine in alcoholic solution.

NP 27 (Norwich)—Liquid containing orthochloromercuriphenol, benzoic and salicylic acid, and propyl paraben.

Sopronol Powder (Wyeth)—Contains sodium propionate, sodium caprylate, and zinc propionate.

Sulfur 1% and Salicylic Acid 1% Ointment (Various Manufacturers)—Contains 1% each of sulfur and salicylic acid as either an ointment or lotion.

Tinactin Cream (Schering)—Contains tolnaftate 1% with butylated hydroxytoluene (a preservative) and titanium dioxide in an emulsified base. Also solution and powder. Synthetic fungicide, reported to be nonsensitizing.

Whitfield's Ointment—Half Strength (Various Manufacturers)—Contains 6% benzoic acid and 3% salicylic acid in an ointment base. A Whitfield's lotion has the same ingredients in the same strength in 70% alcohol and is often preferable.

WARTS

DEFINITION

Warts are horny growths on the skin, ranging from pinhead-sized to pea-sized, either the color of the skin or darker, and they may be single or multiple.

CAUSE

An infection with the polyoma virus.

DISCUSSION AND CAUTIONS

Warts have figured prominently in folk tales. Evil old women, witches, bad dwarfs, magicians, are all reputed and pictured to have warts on their faces. There is probably a rich anthropological or folk literature as to the role of warts in different nations and cultures.

The folk remedies are probably as many as the warts they purport to treat. They include such remedies as Tom Sawyer's wart water, which is found in tree stumps after a rain; frogs, which are reputed both to bring on and to cure warts; applications of copper pennies, which at least have the advantage of economy. One prominent Cincinnati dermatologist has his children patients make a drawing of their hands with the warts in place. They send him the drawings. He burns them. Frequently the warts disappear, he reports.

Warts sometimes disappear by themselves with no apparent reason. Medical treatment of warts is surgical, by excision of the growth or freezing by liquid nitrogen. Other medical treatment includes application of podophyllin, which is extremely irritating but often effective. An older method has been application of corrosive acids, which raise a considerable inflammation, but this is obviously unsuitable when the wart is on the face.

All this means that warts should not be self-treated. There are two reasons: (a) the treatment, such as it is, requires medical attention; (b) the few over-the-counter remedies are needlessly irritating, simply because they are not effective. Do not use them.

In the Middle Ages warts were cured by incantations. If you use that method and are successful in getting rid of warts, you will have one advantage: incantations are not irritating nor inflammatory to the skin.

DANDRUFF

DEFINITION

Dandruff is a disorder of the skin, usually the scalp, characterized by itching and a profusion of falling dry scales.

CAUSE

Probably a familial predisposition to oily scalp, but it may be due to a hormonal condition where oil secretion is involved, modified by nutritional factors or tension.

DISCUSSION AND CAUTIONS

Dandruff remedies do not remedy dandruff. But they remove the flakes or scales. Dandruff will form again. Certain preparations containing antiseptics, not necessarily shampoos, are also available to retard the reappearance of the dandruff flakes. It is questionable whether reliance can be placed on them, though antiseptic preparations are logically useful. However, shampooing to assure cleanliness of the scalp is the best approach to the control of dandruff. At present, control is the best that can be achieved.

INGREDIENTS

Selenium sulfide shampoo is the most effective for dandruff control. Also useful are the additives to shampoo, such as detergents or antiseptics as salicylic acid, sulfur, resorcin, hexachlorophene, or diiodohydroxyquin. Salicylic acid softens the skin debris (flakes) and facilitates removal by shampooing. The principal objective is to keep the scalp clean.

However, bear in mind that a shampoo remains in contact with the scalp for a very short time.

Even sulfur and salicylic acid in a shampoo do not remain in contact long enough to exert a substantial effect. The best means of using these substances is to apply them and allow them to remain in contact with the scalp for varying lengths of time (use caution against undue irritation). Then use a shampoo to cleanse the scalp. This may be done once to twice a week, depending on the reformation of flakes.

Cetyltrimethyl ammonium bromide, stearyldimethylbenzyl ammonium chloride, polyoxyethylene lauryl ether, hexachlorophene, alkyldimethyl benzyl ammonium chloride (benzalkonium chloride), and lauryl isoquinolinium bromide are surface-active agents (wetting agents or detergents) and antiseptics.

Zinc pyrithione is a fungicide and antiseptic owing its effect to a sulfur and zinc combination. Triclocarban is an antiseptic. Both products are active in a soap combination.

The following ingredients are surface-active agents and emulsifiers, and some are antiseptic: polyoxyethylene nonyl phenol, polyoxyethylenelauryl alcohol (Brij), and lauryl isoquinolinium bromide.

Entsufon is the trade name for sodium octylphenoxyethoxyethyl ether sulfonate, a surface-active agent.

Among the listing of the following products some are shampoos; others are applications after shampoo as antiseptic lotions or hair grooming preparations. All shampoos obviously contain surface-active agents or detergents.

If Your Need Is for a Product Against Dandruff:

Look for Products Containing the Following Ingredients:

- Selenium sulfide
- Salicylic acid
- Sulfur
- Hexachlorophene
- Benzalkonium chloride
- Coal tar

NAMES OF PRODUCTS

AGAINST DANDRUFF

Breck One (American Cyanamid)—Contains zinc pyrithione.

Ceta-Tar Shampoo (Alcon)—Contains 2% salicylic acid, 0.2% benzalkonium chloride, coal tar in detergent base, and 13% alcohol.

Double Danderine (Glenbrook/Sterling)—Contains alkyldimethyl benzyl ammonium chloride and 9% alcohol. Not a shampoo, but a lotion for use after shampoo.

Enden Dandruff Shampoo (Helene Curtis)—Contains hexachlorophene.

Head & Shoulders Dandruff Shampoo (Procter & Gamble)—Contains zinc pyrithione.

Ionil T Dandruff Shampoo (Owen)—Contains salicylic acid 2%, coal tar, benzalkonium chloride 0.2%, and alcohol 13%.

Mazon Medicated Shampoo (Thayer)—Contains coal tar solution 2.5% and hexachlorophene 0.5%.

Meted Antidandruff Shampoo (Texas)—Contains sulfur 3%, salicylic acid 2%, and triclocarban 1%.

Rinse Away After-Shampoo Rinse (Alberto-Culver)—Contains benzalkonium chloride and lauryl isoquinolinium bromide 0.8%. Lotion after shampooing.

Scadan Scalp Lotion (Dome)—Contains cetyltrimethyl ammonium bromide 1% and stearyldimethylbenzyl ammonium chloride 0.1%. Lotion after shampooing.

Sebaquin Dandruff Shampoo (Summers)—Contains diiodohydroxyquin 3% in lanolin fraction.

Sebb (Max Factor)—Contains benzethonium chloride, *N*-trichloromethylmercapto-4-cyclohexene-1,2-dicarboximide, and alcohol 19%.

Sebucare Medicated Scalp Lotion (Westwood)—Contains polyoxyethylenelauryl ether 5%, salicylic acid 2%, and hexachlorophene 0.5%. For grooming after shampooing.

Sebulex Antiseborrheic Shampoo (Westwood)—Contains sulfur 2%, salicylic acid 2%, and hexachlorophene 1%.

Sebutone Antiseborrheic Tar Shampoo (Westwood)—Contains coal tar 0.5%, lanolin fraction, hexachlorophene 1%, sulfur 2%, and salicylic acid 2%.

Selsun Shampoo, Blue (Abbott)—Contains selenium sulfide 1%.

Subdue Dandruff Shampoo (Alberto-Culver)—No ingredients listed.

Sulfur-8 Medicated Shampoo (Pharmaco)—Contains hexachlorophene.

ACNE

DEFINITION

Acne is an inflammation of the skin characterized by oiliness, pimples, and pustules; it usually occurs in both sexes during adolescence.

CAUSE

The hormonal development before and during puberty is presumably the cause. However, there may be individual or familial predisposition to the development of acne.

DISCUSSION AND CAUTIONS

Acne occurs at the time it hurts most, in adolescence, when youngsters are most eager to match or exceed their peers. It is a skin condition that does psychic damage, figuratively speaking. It should not be waved away by adults with the cheery but vacuous "You'll outgrow it." While youngsters frequently (but not invariably) do outgrow it, they may carry with them to later life the results of what acne may have done to their self-esteem, personality development, or self-confidence. What infectious diseases are to childhood, acne is to adolescence. It is a disease of puberty.

Make no mistake about it: acne can be as distressing to boys as to girls. And the psychic trauma that a moderate case of acne can induce can be as damaging as an unrequited love affair.

Adolescence is a time of considerable stress, psychologically as well as physically. We shall touch only on the physical aspect. In adolescence there is an increase in kind and quantity of metabolic activity during the process of growing up. And with sexual maturation there is a hormonal upheaval. Boys and girls becoming men and women pay the price of the side effect of that maturation. One of them is acne.

Indeed, you can tell your youngsters that acne is the sign that they are maturing sexually, blooming into men and women, and that eunuchs do not get acne. While we think it is well to point that out, we believe that it is an empty solace. Parents should understand that if youngsters do not respond to the empty solace they offer, it does not mean that the youngsters are recalcitrant.

Acne is the pregnancy of adolescence. Youngsters, especially girls, can be expected to react with emotional anarchy to the cheerful encouragement of parents who do not have acne. (And the cheer from parents who are scarred from adolescent acne can be even worse.) We really do not know what you can tell your youngsters to lighten the weight of the cross of adolescence. Just try to be perceptive and compassionate. You may be clobbered anyway, but at least you will not add to the youngster's burden.

A moderate, and surely a severe, case of acne should be handled by a dermatologist. The products available over-the-counter without a prescription are of three kinds: (a) those that merely cover a blemish, (b) those that have ingredients such as hexachlorophene, sulfur or salicylic acid which do something, and (c) combinations of the foregoing. But these products are not a treatment; they are a temporary stopgap. They may be helpful for special occasions or between visits to the dermatologist.

The objective in handling acne is not only to make the blemishes less conspicuous but to prevent permanent scarring. The scars are more than skin-deep: they affect the adult's feeling of self-esteem. Visualize a woman who has appreciable acne scars on her back. She avoids the beach because no bathing suit can cover them. And acne scars on the face, which is exposed every day, often raise havoc with her and her interpersonal relations.

While acne cannot be cleared up in a week, many steps can be taken by the youngsters to lessen the skin trauma and at least not to make the acne worse.

The first is cleanliness of the skin. In acne, the oil glands are overactive. In old age they are underactive, leading to dry skin. The use of detergents several times a day to emulsify and wash away the oil is not helpful because the glands secrete more oil in about an hour. Cleanliness is helped, however, by regular use of one of the skin cleansers containing hexachlorophene or by soap containing hexachlorophene.

One of the problems in acne is that oil accumulates when the pores are plugged. It is important to keep them unplugged, both by skin cleanliness and by *gentle* removal of blackheads. The emphasis is on *gentle*. Care should be taken that no injury to the skin results from blackhead removal, to prevent infection or the development of large pores, which become a lifelong heritage of careless and energetic blackhead removal. Let a dermatologist show you how to do it.

Cleanliness can also be aided by frequent and careful use of aluminum oxide paste (this is *not* aluminum hydroxide) as directed by a dermatologist. That paste contains abrasive particles of aluminum oxide in a soap or detergent base and can be washed off after gently massaging into the skin.

The acne pimples are little pus centers. The objective is to clean them and to prevent them from becoming larger. This is helped by cleansing and gentle handling, as shown you by a dermatologist. Do not handle or squeeze acne idly! If you remember that acne is an inflammation of the skin in which the fat-secreting glands are involved, you will remember to exercise caution in handling. *Do not squeeze them! Avoid spreading the infection!*

Acne is not a purely local phenomenon, but is triggered by the hormonal upheaval that adolescence represents. Therefore it is clear that systemic dysfunctions and nutrition have a role in it. Unfortunately, no simple dietary measure is known to make acne better.

Certain foods, such as chocolate, nuts, cola drinks, coffee, and perhaps dairy products, are believed to make it worse. But a broad and rigid dietary restriction is probably a worse mistake; adequate nutrition is necessary during adolescence to meet the metabolic needs of growth and to satisfy the proverbial large appetites of adolescence. How the prohibition of coffee and cola drinks—a hallmark of adolescent indulgence—can be put into effect, we frankly do not know. But surely, the use of skim milk instead of whole milk is no sacrifice, and can be done with comparatively little trouble.

Fried or fatty foods should be avoided, not because we know of a direct relationship between acne and fatty foods, but because added fat may possibly produce more oil on the skin.

One of the symptoms of intoxication with certain drugs is skin outbreaks such as boils. Among them are iodides and bromides. Merely for that reason, and not because we know of a direct relationship, adolescents should avoid iodides (iodine-containing drugs) and bromides. Iodides are found in certain cough mixtures and are often used in treating diseases of the thyroid. Iodized salt also contains iodine, but the amount of iodine therein is merely a trace.

Bromides are sedatives. They are used much less frequently now. But a small amount of potassium bromide is found in Bromo Seltzer. It serves a logical purpose there, but adolescents should use another analgesic on the rare occasions they need one for headache or menstrual pain.

As a general principle other drugs should be avoided, if feasible, because it is not known what can make acne worse. Direct sunlight is fine for the adolescent skin, and for the acne.

But too much of a good thing can spell sunburn. *This should be especially avoided in acne areas,* as infection can occur or spread.

As mentioned previously, adolescence is also a time of emotional stress. In fact, such stress can well be a factor in emotional maturation. You cannot wrap adolescents in cotton wool to protect them, even if they were to let you! But adolescents should realize that both interpersonal contact or world conditions they hope to reform are fueled by emotion.

Is emotion tied up to secretion of oil by the skin? Indirectly, yes, for emotion increases metabolic activity. Increased metabolic activity accelerates all body functions, including secretion of oil by the skin, and this can make acne worse. Each person must find and strike the balance between emotional upheaval and apathy.

INGREDIENTS

Sulfur, salicylic acid, resorcinol, and hexachlorophene serve good purposes in acne preparations.

Sulfur, salicylic acid, and resorcinol remove skin debris; in fact they peel skin in strong concentration. However, they are not, and should not be, of such a concentration in over-the-counter acne preparations. They carry another advantage: they stimulate local circulation, which accounts for the slight reddening of skin. They are also antiseptic but are basically used for their skin softening (keratoplastic) action. (Resorcinol and resorcin are synonyms.)

Benzoic acid and hexachlorophene are antiseptic, protecting against infection. Phenol (carbolic acid), camphor, menthol, oil of eucalyptus or clove, and thymol are also antiseptic, but in the proportions used they are not as effective as benzoic acid or hexachlorophene. Menthol does give a cooling sensation which may be a comfort if the skin is hot. But when the skin is hot enough to be inflamed and uncomfortable, the problem is more than superficial. Menthol in that case would be a detriment rather than a help, for it would give false security that all is well. It is not. To prevent the spread of infection you should let your dermatologist decide what measures to use.

Boric acid is among the useless antiseptics in acne. In fact, saturated solutions of boric acid often develop mold in the bottle!

Polyoxyethylene lauryl ether (no relationship to ether used in anesthesia), also known as Brij, and polyoxyethylene sorbitan monooleate, also known as Tween 80 or polysorbate 80, are emulsifying agents, making the oil secretion on the skin soluble so that it can be washed away easily. They are also good additions to acne remedies.

Among surface-active agents or detergents, some of which are also antiseptic: polyoxyethylenenonyl phenol, polyoxyethylene lauryl ether, and Entsufon (sodium octylphenoxyethoxyethyl ether sulfonate).

Among mild abrasives, to facilitate a cleansing or scouring action, are polyethylene beads or granules and aluminum oxide particles.

For cleansing in acne do not use oils. They add to the problem. Solutions containing alcohol or small proportions of acetone (5% to 15%) are much better. The hexachlorophene-containing soaps are preferable for daily use. If used sporadically they are less effective. Used regularly, two or three times a day, they build up an antiseptic layer.

The most efficient cleansing of the skin is effected by the use of certain detergents. They remove oil and grime more efficiently than soap. However, to prevent excessive drying effects, lanolin derivatives are added. A small amount of liquid petrolatum (mineral oil) also overcomes, in some measure, the drying effect of the detergents. However, avoid excess use.

For its antiseptic as well as a cleansing effect, hexachlorophene is used broadly and successfully in concentrations up to 3%.

Skin cleansers are especially necessary in conjunction with the self-treatment of acne.

Other ingredients used infrequently, sodium thiosulfate owes its effect to sulfur, but sulfur is more direct. Colloidal sulfur means sulfur subdivided in ultrafine particles (colloidal). If truly colloidal, it may be preferable to the regular precipitated sulfur, though that variety is commonly used quite effectively.

Substances that are used in the vehicle of acne preparations are titanium dioxide, bentonite, or kaolin, often slightly tinted to approximate the color of skin. These substances are not antiseptic, nor detergent, but merely act as a needed cosmetic cover.

We spoke of certain ingredients, like sulfur, that "stimulate" skin. *Stimulation is merely another word for irritation!* If you stimulate skin sufficiently, it is irritated. Stimulation and irritation are differences of degree, not of kind. If irritation develops or persists, your dermatologist should handle the problem. Don't use an over-the-counter acne preparation.

Adolescents are particulary sensitive to slight changes in the skin—hue, texture, elevation. Girls, even those without acne, commonly examine their face in a magnifying mirror in the morning to assess the ravages the night may have brought. They often see fancied blemishes.

Naturally, real if temporary blemishes can send them into a near-panic. One of these is a cold sore or fever sore (herpes simplex). Usually it occurs on the lips. Compound tincture of benzoin is probably better for treatment than lip pomades.

Compound tincture of benzoin is an alcoholic solution of water-insoluble gums. When applied to the cold sore, or in fact anywhere on the skin, it seals that spot with an impervious cover. While it does not do away with a cold sore, it reduces some of its discomfort. Then, the site on which the compound tincture of benzoin has been applied can be covered with a spot of powder to reduce its conspicuousness.

If Your Need Is for a Product Against Acne:

Look for Products Containing the Following Ingredients:

- Resorcinol
- Sulfur
- Salicylic acid
- Benzoic acid
- Hexachlorophene

Benzalkonium chloride
Detergents, as
polyoxyethylene lauryl ether or Entsufon
Abrasives, as
aluminum oxide particles

NAMES OF PRODUCTS

AGAINST ACNE

Acne Aid Lotion (Stiefel)—Contains 10% sulfur and 10% alcohol in a lotion base.

Acne-Dome Medicated Cleanser (Dome)—Contains colloidal sulfur, salicylic acid, and hexachlorophene.

Acnomel Acne Cake (Smith Kline & French)—Contains resorcinol 1%, sulfur 4%, and hexachlorophene 0.25%. (Also available as a cream.)

Alphacene Skin Cleanser and Acne Treatment Combination (Doak)—Skin cleanser contains hexachlorophene. Acne treatment contains colloidal sulfur, resorcin, and hexachlorophene.

Brasivol Scrub Cleanser for Acne (Stiefel)—Contains:
Fine—38% aluminum oxide particles and 1% hexachlorophene.
Medium—52% aluminum oxide particles and 1% hexachlorophene.
Rough—65% aluminum oxide particles and 1% hexachlorophene, in a detergent paste.

Clear Complexion Gel for Acne (Jergens)—Contains hexachlorophene, benzyl alcohol 1%, allantoin, menthol, alcohol 38%, and detergent.

Clearasil Medicated Cream (Vick)—Contains sulfur, resorcinol, hexachlorophene, bentonite, and alcohol 10%.

Clearasil Medicated Lotion (Vick)—Contains sulfur, resorcinol, hexachlorophene, bentonite, and alcohol 13%.

Clearasil Medicated Stick (Vick)—Contains sulfur, resorcinol, hexachlorophene, bentonite, and alcohol.

Fostril Acne Drying Lotion (Westwood)—Contains polyoxyethylene lauryl ether 6%, hexachlorophene 1%, and colloidal sulfur 2%.

Freshstart Acne Medicine (Colgate-Palmolive)—Contains polyoxyethylenenonyl phenol, hexachlorophene, allantoin, isopropanol 23%, and alcohol 21% (total alcohol is 44%).

HyperpHaze (Colgate-Palmolive)—Contains hexachlorophene 3%, ethoxylated lanolin, carbamide, and light liquid petrolatum.

Komed Acne Lotion (Barnes-Hind)—Contains sodium thiosulfate 8%, salicylic acid 2%, resorcinol 2%, isopropanol 25%, alumina, menthol, and camphor.

Microsyn Acne Lotion (Syntex)—Contains sodium thiosulfate 8%, salicylic acid 2%, resorcinol 2%, and alcohol 25% in a colloidal alumina lotion.

Pernox Lathering Cleanser (Westwood)—Contains granules of polyethylene, sulfur 2%, salicylic acid 1.5%, and hexachlorophene 1% in a wetting agent.

pHisoac Cream (Winthrop)—Contains colloidal sulfur 6%, resorcinol 1.5%, and hexachlorophene 0.3%.

pHisodan Medicated Shampoo (Winthrop)—Contains precipitated sulfur 5%, sodium salicylate 0.5%, hexachlorophene 3%, with Entsufon, lanolin cholesterols, and petrolatum.

pHisoderm Antibacterial Skin Cleanser (Winthrop)—Contains Entsufon, lanolin cholesterols, petrolatum, and 3% hexachlorophene. (The difference among the following three pHisoderm products may be only a difference of proportion of Entsufon and petrolatum; no quantities listed on label.)

pHisoderm Dry Type (Winthrop)—Contains Entsufon, lanolin cholesterols, and petrolatum.

pHisoderm Oily Type Sudsing Detergent (Winthrop)—Contains Entsufon, lanolin cholesterols, and petrolatum.

pHisoderm Regular Type Sudsing Detergent (Winthrop)—Contains Entsufon, lanolin cholesterols, and petrolatum.

pHisoHex Antibacterial Skin Cleanser (Winthrop)—Contains Entsufon and hexachlorophene.

Polybrade Acne Cleanser (Texas)—Contains fine, polyethylene granules in detergent base.

Propa-P.H. (Bio Products)—Contains benzoic acid, boric acid, thymol, eucalyptol, oil of thyme, and alcohol 28%.

Proseca (Westwood)—Contains polyoxyethylene lauryl ether 3%, sulfur 4%, hexachlorophene 1%, with surface-active agents.

SAStid Cream—Acne Therapeutic Wash (Stiefel)—Contains sulfur 1.6%, salicylic acid 1.6%, and hexachlorophene 0.8%.

SAStid (AL) Cream—Acne Scrub Cleanser (Stiefel)—Contains sulfur 1.6%, salicylic acid 1.6%, hexachlorophene 0.8%, and aluminum oxide particles 20% in surface-active agents.

Tackle Medicated Clear Gel (Colgate-Palmolive)—No ingredients listed.

Thera-Blem Cream (Noxell)—Contains hexachlorophene, sulfur, resorcinol, phenol (less than 0.5%), menthol, camphor, clove oil, and eucalyptus oil.

Therapads Plus (Fuller)—Pads saturated with 70% alcohol and 1.5% salicylic acid with detergent.

Tyrosum Skin Cleanser for Acne (Summers)—Contains polysorbate-80 2%, acetone 10%, and isopropanol 50%.

Xerac Gel (Person & Covey)—Contains sulfur 4%, hexachlorophene 1%, and alcohol 44% in a plastic gel.

Young People Medicated Moist Towelettes (Young)—Contains hexachlorophene, polyoxyethylene lauryl ether, menthol, isopropanol 15%, and alcohol 15%.

Zephiran Spray (Winthrop)—Contains benzalkonium chloride 0.13% and alcohol 24%.

SKIN LOTIONS

Lotions are fluid preparations by means of which many substances may be applied to the skin. They are especially useful when it is desired to cover a surface with a residual film, or when ointments should not be used for some reason, or are inconvenient to use. Lotions may be classified on a basis of their physical characteristics as (1) shake-lotions, (2) emulsions, and (3) solutions. The comments made here about lotions frequently apply as well to other preparations used on the skin.

GENERAL ACTION OF LOTIONS

Generally, the effect of lotions is superficial and topical. But many factors and influences may exert an effect different from that which is intended; that effect may be an undesirable one. Lotions, particularly shake-lotions, are intended for topical effect. They are especially suitable in superficial skin irritations and may be applied over a large portion of the body, provided they do not contain substances that are absorbable from their vehicle and when absorbed give rise to systemic effects. An example is a lotion containing phenol (carbolic acid).

The pharmacological action of lotions depends on two factors: (a) the nature of the so-called vehicle and (b) the nature of the so-called active ingredient. The nature of the vehicle influencing the effect of lotions may be of primary importance. With this concept in mind, a vehicle cannot be considered to be inactive. The physical assistance that a vehicle confers usually plays as active a part as the so-called active ingredient used in a lotion for its therapeutic effect.

By way of illustration: therapeutic additives, for example, salicylic acid and boric acid in water as a vehicle, make up a bacteriostatic lotion. But the same therapeutic additives in a 50% alcoholic solution as a vehicle compose a skin peeling and mildly fungicidal lotion. The vehicle has changed the function of the same active ingredients present in the same quantity.

The above illustrations suggest another factor, an obvious one, with respect to the proportion of the therapeutic additive. The same therapeutic additive, salicylic acid, in strengths of 1% to 3% may be germicidal. But in a 5% to 25% strength it may be skin softening (keratoplastic) or skin peeling or skin destroying (keratolytic) as well.

Lotions, in contradistinction to ointments or pastes, are highly diffusive. They spread efficiently, seep and enter into the cracks, crevices, natural folds such as those between the fingers, and acquired folds such as wrinkles.

APPLICATION

Lotions are applied directly to the skin, not by using gauze or other textile material saturated with lotion. The application of textile materials wetted with lotion vitiates the very purpose a lotion is designed to serve—complete and intimate contact of lotion and site on the skin.

If a site to which a lotion has been applied must be bandaged, the bandaging material should be saturated with the lotion before being applied to the site to which the lotion has been previously applied. The reason lies in the necessity of preventing the bandaging material from absorbing the lotion.

SENSORY EFFECT

Most water-based lotions or those containing alcohol and water are cooling owing to the evaporation of the solution or vehicle—a simple physical principle. Lotions are cooling in direct relation to their vapor pressure: the more rapidly a lotion evaporates, the more quickly it cools the skin. For example, ethyl chloride, which is used as a local anesthetic by spraying on the skin and evaporates almost instantaneously, cools extremely quickly; continuous application and evaporation cools the site to the point of freezing it. Hydroalcoholic lotions cool very efficiently. Aqueous lotions cool reasonably satisfactorily.

On the other hand, lotions containing oils do not cool efficiently. The presence of even 1% of oil reduces the cooling ability of a lotion out of proportion to the influence that such a small amount of oil would be expected to exert. The reason is apparent: despite the evaporation of the aqueous or hydroalcoholic portion of a lotion, the film of oil left on the site covers the skin with a *liquid glove,* or film, which retains heat. In fact, additional applications will *increase heat retention,* for the more lotion that is applied, the greater the oily residue on the skin. Oil-in-water emulsions are an exception, for though they contain oil, the oil content is emulsified so that the water phase is predominant and the oil film is not continuous. Such an exception does not apply to water-in-oil emulsions.

There is an *apparent* exception to the heat-retaining effect of an oil lotion—namely, a lotion containing oil and menthol. Such a lotion does not leave a feeling of heat at the site owing to the sensory cooling effect of menthol. Nonetheless, that cooling effect is only a seeming one; the lack of sensation of heat and congestion is the response of the cutaneous nerve endings to menthol. The heat in the tissues is not reduced. What little reduction of heat that does occur in a lotion containing oil and menthol is probably due to the effect on skin circulation of the stimulus offered by menthol to the cutaneous nerve endings. But another factor, the rubefacient effect of menthol, obscures the picture.

CONTACT WITH LESION

In the absence of oil or fatty materials, the evaporation of a lotion commonly leaves the therapeutic additive in intimate contact with the lesion or the site of application. Upon evaporation of the vehicle, the therapeutic additive is usually left on the site *in its full strength,* provided it is not more volatile than the vehicle. For that reason, lotions, particularly aqueous or hydroalcoholic lotions, and especially those which do not contain glycerine or oils, are vastly superior to ointments or pastes in bringing to the lesion the full effect of the therapeutic additive. The effect of ointments or pastes is limited to the extremely narrow zone of contact between lesion and the first molecular layer of ointment.

Another situation in which lotions function more efficiently than ointments is on sites that are particularly hairy—i.e., in the armpit, in the groin, and often on the chest or back. A more efficient contact between medication and lesion on hairy sites is established by a lotion than by an ointment. In that light, the claim that a particular ointment is especially suitable for hairy areas is often without foundation. Whereas it may be true that a given ointment may wash out from a hairy area more efficiently, it is not more suitable if it has the melting point and viscosity of an ointment, since it does not contact the lesion as well as a lotion.

PREPARE SKIN

Certain acts preparatory to the application of a lotion assure optimum effect. For example, the application of an aqueous lotion to a site on which an ointment has been previously applied is unwise, as the ointment residue creates a seal, inhibiting contact between lotion and lesion. In such cases it is desirable to wash the site, if not contraindicated, with rubbing alcohol in order to remove residue of medication, grime, sebum, etc. Or a suitable synthetic aqueous detergent can be employed for that purpose.

OTHER EFFECTS OF LOTIONS

Astringent lotions are used to arrest secretions or to control inflammation. They exert their effect by the precipitation of tissue protein. Though witch hazel is the traditional astringent lotion, more effective astringent lotions contain a higher proportion of alcohol, or alum, or zinc salts.

At times a superficial stimulating effect in certain stages of acne is desirable. For that purpose either tar, sulfur, benzoic or salicylic acids, or resorcin, or their combinations are used. The effect of such lotions is keratoplastic and, in high concentration, keratolytic.

Antiseptic lotions have their limitations due either to poor solubility of most antiseptic substances in aqueous solutions or, if they are soluble, to the irritating effects of the antiseptics themselves. However, bacterial inhibition may be accomplished by the use of hexachlorophene or other suitable agents in lotions.

With the continuing development of pharmaceutical preparations due to newer synthetic materials, shake-lotions may not be the simple suspensions they were thought to be. For example, the addition of fat or oil to a shake-lotion may render it an emulsion. Emulsions have entirely different pharmacological bases and therefore usually different therapeutic effects. Also, the absorption characteristics of a shake-lotion may be changed by the addition of nonfat substances as the polyethylene glycols, surface-active agents as sodium lauryl sulfates, benzalkonium chloride, lanolin alcohols, etc. These substances are frequently added to increase the elegance, homogeneity, or appearance of shake-lotions. There is nothing wrong with the use of these substances *per se.* But such preparations are not shake-lotions in effect.

INGREDIENTS

The Federal Food, Drug and Cosmetic Act requires the listing on the labels of the *quantity* and *kind* of active ingredients or products restricted to sale on prescription. It requires the listing of only the *kind* of active ingredients of those products not labeled with the prescription legend and therefore those which can be sold without a prescription. (An exception resides in certain drugs such as mercury, arsenic, alcohol, etc., in which event the *quantity* as well as *kind* of ingredient must be given in any case.) The act does not require the listing of inactive ingredients.

OTHER LOTIONS

But it does not mean that shake-lotions—those which show a separation of solid and liquid, as calamine lotion—are the only lotions available. The term *lotion* may also connote a clear liquid or a milky liquid, common to hand lotions used for cosmetic purposes.

GENERAL ARTICLES ON TOPICS OF HEALTH AND DISEASE

ABOUT SIDE EFFECTS

The phrase *side effect* is often regarded as if it were a dirty word. We should, however, reexamine what it means in the context in which it applies to what we've been discussing in this book.

A side effect is commonly understood as an untoward, secondary effect from a drug that is taken for a particular purpose. For example, antihistamines are taken to control the symptoms of hay fever. However, they have a *side effect:* they can produce drowsiness. This is an effect that has nothing to do with hay fever and is usually not sought.

In many drugs, however, especially in drugs that are on prescription, there may be side effects that are indeed serious and often dictate that further administration of the drug should cease. That is the reason that the label "side effects" has become a *slur* label.

Yet, certain side effects of a drug can be utilized to advantage. Again take the example of the antihistamines: The drowsiness-producing effect is useful when relaxation and sleep induction are sought. In fact, this is used in over-the-counter sedative preparations. Of course, this does not mean that the drowsiness-producing effect of antihistamines when used to control symptoms of hay fever, or as an ingredient in preparations for control of cough and cold, should be ignored. Since they produce such side effects, tasks requiring alertness or care as to safety should not be undertaken when using the drugs.

Penicillin is frequently considered to have a side effect—i.e., causing skin outbreaks or other allergic conditions. This is really not a side effect, but a reaction of people sensitive to penicillin. That is not an intrinsic quality of the drug.

There is another effect called a side effect which is not one. An example is the hemorrhage that may be caused when an excessive amount of anticoagulant is used. Anticoagulants prevent blood clots, since they reduce the coagulability of the blood. An exaggeration of that is hemorrhage. In other words, coagulability of the blood can be reduced to such an extent that it "thins" blood so excessively that it "bleeds" through the tissues. But reduction of coagulability is exactly what was originally sought. That effect of anticoagulants has merely gone much farther than originally intended, and hemorrhage is an *extension* of the effect of the drug. The occurrence of hemorrhage as a result of taking anticoagulant drugs is therefore properly called an *extension effect,* not a side effect.

Over-the-counter drugs also often have side effects which are not sought. For example, belladonna is a component in some tablets used to treat the symptoms of the common cold. The reason is based on one of the effects of belladonna—drying up secretions. For a runny nose that is helpful. But belladonna has a side effect that is not looked for. In large doses it can produce a rapid heartbeat or palpitations. The labels usually warn the user that when that occurs, the further taking of a product containing belladonna should be discontinued. Sometimes the labels call it palpitations, at other times tachycardia. In this context it means the same thing.

However, the side effects of drugs that are available over-the-counter without prescription are not believed to be of the degree of, or as threatening as, those of drugs sold on prescription only. In fact, this is one consideration that figures prominently in the decisions of the FDA as to whether a product is or is not suitably safe for over-the-counter sale.

For that reason, among others, read the labels completely. They are both safety and informational devices. Most reputable firms pay particular attention to be sure that the cautions and warnings on side effects are clearly given on the labels.

It is well known that some medications which, when taken by themselves are reasonably safe, become unsafe and often dangerous when taken with other medicines. This is an important phenomenon. However, when this phenomenon occurs it is found in prescription drugs, not in over-the-counter remedies available without prescription. In the rare instances that this may apply to over-the-counter drugs, we have made clear mention of it in the text. An example was when we cautioned the reader not to take aspirin when he is taking anticoagulants prescribed by his physician.

THE SKIN AS SIGNAL OF DISEASE

Skin lesions are commonly treated for cosmetic reasons or for the discomfort they may produce, such as itching. At times, however, skin lesions actually serve a purpose. They warn of a developing systemic disease; in some of them skin lesions are one of the first signs. The most widely known of such signs is Koplik's spots, which appear in the mouth before the general appearance of the spots of measles. A skin lesion due to, or heralding, an internal disease is even given a special name. It is called an *exanthesis.*

Among the various lesions of the skin, any of which may be signs of a constitutional or systemic disease, are itching, hives, little hard nodules, change in skin temperature or color, blisters, and rashes.

SKIN COLOR

A change in skin color may be a harbinger of an internal disease. We are talking of a change in the color of the skin over a large area of the body, such as yellow pigmentation. That this may suggest the development of jaundice is well known, or it may occur when jaundice due to liver disease has already developed. Equally well known is the bronzing of skin due to Addison's disease, a disease of the adrenal glands. Less well known but of grave importance is the discoloration of the skin, either in large patches or virtually over all of the body, which at times presages visceral cancer or Hodgkin's disease before any other symptoms are apparent. Pigmentation of the skin can also occur due to an anomaly in the assimilation of nutrients, as in the malabsorption syndrome.

A color change that is limited in area is purpura, due to hemorrhage under the skin. These purpuras are often signs of constitutional or systemic disturbances, or they may be prophetic, signifying an impending systemic condition. Purpuras, or purple patches, may suggest a fulminating condition in the body and may occur before such diseases as colitis, uremia, leukemia, or ulcerative colitis, among other conditions. While the purpura may disappear, the systemic condition may remain as a troublesome sequel.

ITCHING

Perhaps itching is the most common sign on the skin of an impending systemic disease. Hodgkin's disease, leukemia, visceral cancer, diabetes, thyroid disease, liver disease, or certain blood disturbances are frequently preceded by itching. At other times itching may occur after they develop. Itching due to psychic causes is perhaps equally frequent. This is not at all amazing in view of the fact that the skin, richly supplied with nerve endings, is the target of emotional changes brought on by fear, agitation, frustration, perhaps depression. These changes may be expressed by blanching, blushing, perspiring under tension, and even in the appearance of discrete lesions such as those of lichen planus, which may appear anywhere on the skin, on the mucous membrane, or on the genitals.

BLISTERS

Blisters may also be the first sign of a number of developing internal diseases, as cancer or the malabsorption syndrome.

Pemphigus, a fatal skin disease in some of its variants, has blistering as the principal symptom both in premonitory signs and during the disease state itself. (In fact, the word pemphigus is derived from *pemphix*, a blister in Greek.) Another skin condition characterized by blisters which may be an early sign of a constitutional disease is erythema multiforme, one form of which is an acute inflammatory constitutional disease usually showing its first signs on the skin (as well as on mucous membranes). Ordinarily differential diagnosis in this condition is a difficult problem, and the signs on the skin may aid in the diagnosis.

FLUSHING

One of the common signs of the menopausal syndrome is flushing of the face and neck. This is the result of an imbalance produced by the endocrinological upheaval of the menopause. But sudden transient flushing can be a premonitory sign of another disease, the carcinoid syndrome, produced by a sudden discharge of serotonin from carcinoid tumors. Or sudden flushing can be caused by a pheochromocytoma, a tumor of the adrenal medulla or of other tissues. These tumors secrete epinephrine and cause the sudden upsurge of hypertension.

WHEALS AND HIVES

Hives and wheals are a classic example of an allergic manifestation, a sensitivity to some substance. While the appearance of hives may indeed be a hypersensitivity response to an allergen that is ingested, inhaled or touched, they may be nonetheless a response to an altered protein in the body to which an individual is sensitive. The incipient disease process may alter a particular body protein to which the individual does not ordinarily respond into a protein to which an individual does. Therefore he may break out in hives and wheals, as a direct result of a metabolic change in the body, which may be the signal of an impending disease.

MOUTH

In a parallel fashion the mucous membrane of the mouth, instead of the skin, may also show the first sign of an impending disease. In the mouth, the early warning signs are similar to, though not identical with, those on the skin, i.e., patches, discolorations, increased redness, blisters. An eruption, outbreak, or rash on the skin is called an *exanthem;* an eruption or outbreak in the mouth, or in fact on any mucous membrane, is called an *enanthem.*

Though ulcerations in the mouth, as canker sores or herpes simplex, may be due to poor mouth hygiene or to other local oral conditions, they are not necessarily of local origin. For example, a disease called aphthosis or Behçet's disease—in which there is vascular, muscular, or nervous degeneration—has canker sores of the mouth, as well as lesions on the skin and eyes, as a first sign of the impending disease.

Other diseases of which the first sign may also appear in the mouth are tuberculosis (ulcer) and jaundice (yellow palate); a number of other changes in the mouth may herald some forms of leukemia.

These conditions reaffirm the belief that man is a holistic animal—the wholeness of man as an organism is greater than the sum of his parts. And it also suggests that the tunnel vision that sometimes comes with specialization obscures the sight of the whole organism.

LIVING MATTER TRADES IN ENERGY

DNA and RNA are now magic words. They stand for deoxyribonucleic acid and ribonucleic acid, respectively. You have recently heard a lot about them, and you will hear increasingly more.

They have to do with disease, with health, and in fact with discussions about whether one can artificially modify life by manipulating them. More particularly, through another magic word, ATP (adenosine triphosphate), they deal with energy.

THE POWERHOUSE

All living matter is alive because it trades in energy. Carbohydrates can be likened to materials that compose fuel. But the fuel will not be ignited, and will therefore not liberate the energy required in living, unless certain enzymes and coenzymes, particularly adenosine phosphates, are present to act as "spark plugs" to ignite the fuel. In fact, because of that function of adenosine phosphates they are frequently referred to as "energy-rich phosphates." These substances, igniting the fuel, enable tissues to utilize foodstuff and to convert it to energy for the organism to remain alive and to operate.

Enzymes, amino acids and their proteins, vitamins, minerals, carbohydrates, fats, and other foodstuffs are intimately related in the scheme of body physiology. Any separation of their function is more or less artificial, at times arbitrary, and most frequently done for convenience in order to be able to encompass the numerous fantastically complex changes and interchanges which we call metabolism.

All these materials are important, and some are indispensable. But if one were obliged to single out the most important of the body's functions, it would be its ability to store up and utilize energy. This does not necessarily mean (though it includes) muscular energy for activity, but also the energy used in just sitting still, the energy used while asleep—in fact, the energy of just being alive. ATP is the means of storing and, through its changes, discharging energy.

ENERGY

Energy is necessary to perform all the chemical transformations and detoxifications in the body—the discharge or inactivation of spent or poisonous materials of body metabolism and the utilization of the salubrious materials.

The body is both a chemical factory and a waste disposal plant. We can liken energy in the body to the electrical current in the battery of a motorcar. If the battery is *dead,* no combustion can take place and no combustion products are produced. Though plenty of fuel may be available, no movement of the car can take place.

Where in the body does all this energy storage and discharge take place? Not in any specific organ but in each cell and in the intercellular tissues. (Blood is also considered a tissue.) And this is a continuous process wherein each group of cells acts as a reaction vessel.

Though the reaction is continuous, the rate of reaction varies. The reactions continue during such states as sleep, but at a much lower rate. In the event of starvation or deficiency of some of the vital and essential materials, part of the production line is shut down (lack of raw materials), and the organism is thereby affected. The reason that the organism may appear to be getting along in reasonably good health, even though certain important materials may not be supplied in food or taken as drug, is that the body produces and supplies some of them. Others are not produced by the body and must be taken in as foods or drugs. But any lack of an essential nutrient may interfere with the chain of production farther down the production line.

NUCLEOTIDES

Of the four materials called nucleotides, only adenylic acid carries the ATP potential. The potential energy of ribonucleotides is in the phosphate bonds, but not with the same amount of energy in each bond. Energy is released by the breaking of the bonds, which can be broken at different places with different degrees of energy liberation. In another way of expressing the same concept—oxidative phosphorylation—energy is produced by change in energy-rich bonds. Energy could also be produced as heat, but not with efficient utilization.

IONS

The continuous process of energy formation-discharge-re-formation can go on without certain ions but without them it is labored. The most necessary ion in the process is magnesium. This ion is an activator of certain enzyme systems which are concerned with the separation of phosphates from ATP.

RNA, DNA, MITOCHONDRIA

RNA differs from DNA in the sugars they contain—ribose for RNA and deoxyribose for DNA. Messenger RNA (mRNA) is a carrier or messenger which transmits instructions to the cell directing protein formation.

The complexity of the subject makes any short summary such as this a vast oversimplification. For example, this topic requires a reasonably detailed discussion on the functions in the cell, on the basic operative materials in energy trading, i.e., ribosomes, mitochondria, and chloroplasts. Ribosomes are particles seen only by electron microscope which synthesize the protein after receiving a signal from mRNA. Mitochondria and chloroplasts are the "fuel cells" or power plants; they actually function as energy transformers or *life substances.* Mitochondria are double-walled sacs which carry the enzymes necessary for energy conversion to replenish ATP energy stores. Whereas mitochondria convert chemical energy, chloroplasts (the chlorophyll sacs in plants functioning in photosynthesis) convert light wave energy into ATP energy stores, in the form of bond energy. ATP is the stored energy on which the energy of life processes depends, for all living matter trades in energy.

FEVER

More instances of fever are probably associated with the common cold than any other condition. Yet, a cold is the least serious condition in which fever occurs.

Every rise in body temperature is not fever. Normally, there is a rise in body temperature after a meal, during the process of digestion. Temperature also increases, briefly, after exercise, during ovulation, menstruation and pregnancy, or when the environment is particularly warm and high humidity does not allow the evaporation of moisture. During sleep in the early morning hours (about 3:00 A.M. to 5:00 A.M.) body temperature may be as much as 2° F below normal, reflecting the lowered metabolism and low adrenal activity during sleep. It is highest at 4:00 P.M. to 8:00 P.M. But night workers, by a re-adjustment of their biological rhythm, have a reverse condition—highest temperature during the 3:00 A.M. to 5:00 A.M. period when working, and lowest during the late afternoon or early evening, when asleep.

FLUCTUATIONS

Normal body temperature when awake fluctuates within extremely narrow limits in a given individual, probably by not more than half to one degree Fahrenheit. But the "normal" or standard of 98.6° F (37° C) is merely a working average because individuals vary in their own normal temperature by as much as a degree, or even slightly more. The 98.6° F figure refers to the temperature under the tongue; rectal temperature is usually about one-half degree higher.

Body temperature is the equilibrium between heat production and heat dissipation. Hence, an increased body temperature or fever is basically a greater amount of heat produced than dispersed. The dissipation of heat takes place principally through the skin, which radiates the heat, as well as through the lungs expelled as moist, warm water vapor. Heat is also dissipated by the drinking of cold liquids which, when passed out as warm urine, remove some body heat. But fundamentally, body heat is wondrously regulated or monitored by the hypothalamus, and fever occurs when heat is generated in excess of the body's ability to dissipate it or the hypothalamus to monitor it. An example of a condition associated with fever, wherein the dissipation of heat is far slower than its generation, is heat stroke.

A fever wherein the dissipation of heat is adequate, but the production of heat exceeds the ability to monitor it, can be the result of brain damage. The hypothalamus is involved in the regulation of temperature levels as well as sleep and certain other visceral functions.

HIGH FEVER

Certain diseases may produce high fevers. Examples include those referable to the gastrointestinal system such as salmonella infections or infectious serum hepatitis. High fevers may also be produced by typhoid disease and tropical diseases such as malaria, sprue, or dysentery.

Chronic diseases usually produce prolonged and persistent fevers which are usually not high except in an acute stage. Among these are bronchial diseases, tuberculosis, and rheumatoid arthritis. However, the redness and heat at joints, associated with rheumatoid arthritis (*hot* joints), are not necessarily associated with systemic fever.

A condition recently observed and apparently increasing in frequency is malignant hyperthermia, also called fulminant hyperthermia or *sudden hot fever,* a serious and quite frequently a fatal disease. It may appear after anesthesia. The cause is not infection but a breakdown in energy metabolism (more specifically, an uncoupling of oxidative phosphorylation). To guard against it and in order to recognize it quickly and to treat it, the condition must be borne in mind after anesthesia.

The fevers associated with heart attack as well as cancer are prime examples of fevers due to the destruction of tissue. In the first case, part of the myocardium has been blocked off from nutrition and deterioration sets in. In cancer there is destruction of the invaded tissue.

UP-DOWNS

Fevers can also appear sporadically, wane, and recur. In Hodgkin's disease, a cancer of the lymph tissue, fever usually reflects the recurrence of an active stage of the disease, and abates when there is an arrest of the condition, only to repeat the cycle when the disease is reactivated. Malaria, of course, is the prime example of an intermittent fever—chill, followed by high fever, followed by chill, and the cycle continues. Some inborn errors of metabolism, as familial Mediterranean fever, can also produce a fever that appears and regresses after a day. This is also called episodic fever, which name merely describes the manner of appearance (episode) but does not explain it.

The word *fever* is also part of the name of a number of diseases, probably because fever is one of their most apparent signs. Undulant fever and Malta fever are synonyms for brucellosis; Mediterranean yellow fever or icterohemorrhagic fever is the name for Weil's disease.

Fever activates some of the body's natural defense functions. It is interesting to contemplate that although cancer produces fever due to tissue breakdown, fever may be one of nature's reparative functions, as cancer cells are more sensitive to heat than normal cells.

FEVER AS THERAPY

Fever was induced in the past by intentionally infecting the host with malaria to produce high fever in the treatment of syphilis. But induced-fever therapy became obsolete almost overnight, when penicillin was reported in the 1940s to be the royal remedy for syphilis.

METABOLISM

Drug reactions often produce fever as well as a skin eruption, the reason for the fever often depending on the nature of the drug. Fever associated with an increased pulse rate, accelerated tissue destruction, often also with sleeplessness and restlessness, at times delirium, is not a unitary phenomenon but is the reflection of a number of metabolic events of wide importance. The belief previously held that since fever is not a disease proper but merely a symptom, therefore it need not be treated, is overlooking the profound changes associated with fever. For example, fever increases the metabolic rate, hence increases oxygen demand. And the higher the fever the higher the oxygen demand, which the body may not be able to supply. The belief that was, and may still be, held by some, that the danger lies in the rapid *rate* of temperature rise, not the degree of temperature reached, also appears to be more conjectural than valid. Convulsions, especially in children, occur with high fever, even if it takes days rather than hours to reach its height. In fact, infants and children are much more sensitive to temperature than older people, irrespective of the rate of temperature increase.

Fever could not have been assessed and its progress followed unless done quantitatively by a method that is duplicable and otherwise dependable. In view of the rolé of fever—one of the cornerstones of diagnosis and treatment of disease—it is amazing to note that the fever thermometer was invented only about 100 years ago.

DRUGS

Thyroid substance or extract is known to increase the rate of metabolism, hence oxygen consumption. It would be expected to increase temperature consistent with metabolic acceleration. Paradoxically, it does not cause fever. One reason is that the increased metabolism also accelerates dispersal of heat, which can take place by enhanced perspiration and dilation of the small blood vessels of the skin, which dissipate heat. And there may be other reasons.

ANTIPYRETICS

Fevers are reduced by cooling. One method is cooling the skin by sponging with alcohol and water; the process of evaporation requires heat and thus reduces temperature. This is often done in addition to the use of antipyretics, which dependably reduce temperature.

The antipyretic most widely and also most effectively used is aspirin. Most antipyretics are also analgesics such as salicylamide or APAP (acetaminophen). There is much more to the subject of fever and its treatment than can be handled in this short article.

An amusing sidelight on fever is found in a German book devoted to the subject (*Pharmakotherapie des Fiebers,* 1954), which straightfacedly offers the information that the *principal manifestation of fever is a rise in the body temperature.*

BIOCHEMICAL INTERRELATIONSHIPS

Imagine a world in which all knowledge is thrown helter-skelter into a receptacle—say, a book—where theology adjoins physics and eschatology is treated contiguously with chemistry. Knowledge would be a fragmented set of unrelated events and would offer no basis for its own enlargement or advance. Classification is the first instrument of order. The organization of knowledge is based on order, or upon an orderly classification.

COMPARTMENTS

The urge for classification carries along its caricature, compartmentalization. To classify knowledge is one thing; to sequester it in tight compartments and prevent its cross-fertilization is another.

With the rise of specialization the compartments become tighter, with the resulting loss of communication among the sciences or even among different specialties within the same science. That this is deplorable is obvious, for it is well known that the techniques of one discipline can, and frequently do, enrich another discipline.

BIOCHEMISTRY

The medical sciences are essentially based upon the bedrock of biochemistry. The rise of pharmacology and the interaction and transformation of metabolites in living tissue are due to new techniques and newer concepts in biochemistry. For example, metabolism of hormones, the fate of administered substances, and the synthesis by the body of many materials are based in great measure on the enzymes or coenzymes that aid in, or are indispensable in, the various transformations. This is basically the field of biochemistry.

ELASTICITY

A free interchange of techniques from discipline to discipline can be stimulated by an occasional review of the fundamentals upon which a science is based. It allows one to exchange preconceptions for conceptual thinking, which is the fundamental upon which advances are based. It may help to loosen some rigidity which sets in with time and experience.

Another method by which one can view interrelationships is by a long look into comparative studies as comparative biochemistry. To be sure, the scientist will learn nothing new, either from reviewing fundamentals or from a casual study of the comparative aspects of a science. But suffused with facts, he has often relegated attitudes to the background. Yet, *inventiveness or creativeness springs from attitudes;* they are merely implemented by facts. For that reason many believe that we have too many facts and too few attitudes.

FUNDAMENTALS

A book that can be recommended on this subject is Ernest Baldwin's *The Nature of Biochemistry,** which is intended for the intelligent layman or the undergraduate student. It is to be sure an incomplete presentation of the immense variety in the vast realm of biochemistry, but the research worker does not need a course in biochemistry—he has the facts. However, he can be enriched by a recollection of the fundamentals which spark attitudes.

* *The Nature of Biochemistry,* by E. Baldwin, pp. xiii and 111, Cambridge University Press, New York, 1962.

COMPARATIVE STUDIES

We recall fondly the same author's earlier book of about 40 years ago, Baldwin's *Comparative Biochemistry,* which opened horizons in the understanding of the evolution of animals. There is heuristic value, for example, in the realization that despite various changes in function and adaptation to the environment, the ionic composition of the blood of animals is unusually similar, though their habits, and environment and functions differ. The ionic composition of oceans changed more in millions of years than the ionic composition of blood.

A modern book that enters deeply into such relations and interrelations among living things is Homer Smith's *From Fish to Philosopher.** It details the role of the kidney in the evolution of aquatic to terrestrial animals and describes the role of the kidney in man's current diseases of the heart and blood vessels. Smith, a giant among physiologists, through his comparative studies contributed substantially to the treatment of modern disease.

THE UNCONTROLLABLE VARIABLE

The action of a drug cannot be controlled by thoughts—or can it?

Various procedures are continually being developed to assure controlled studies, especially on drugs, but the most important variable in the system, man and his emotional or mental activities, is virtually uncontrollable. Those aspects in animals are also uncontrollable, despite the fact that the response of animals to drugs is usually extrapolated to man. But mice too, while their emotional and mental activities as such may differ considerably from those of man, also have an intrinsic variable that is not controllable unless it is known and provision in advance is made to correct it.

* *From Fish to Philosopher,* by Homer Smith, pp. xiii and 304, Little, Brown & Co., Boston, 1953.

Another point in this discussion is that while it is well known that drugs can affect an emotional state, it must not be overlooked that the reverse also occurs: the state of mind or emotion can affect the action of a drug.

PHYSICAL–EMOTIONAL

In the past we indulged in that comfortable feeling that a sharp separation could be made between what is physical and what is emotional. It was a comfort because something physical can be identified, measured, duplicated and otherwise classified, while something emotional is considered to be unpredictable, unmeasurable. The latter uncertainty gives rise to discomfort. As science grew, certain canons of behavior were developed. One of those is the scientific method, which has rigid requirements against which the adequacy of a scientific development is measured.

Methods of experimentation in medicine and evaluation of drugs then became more rigid and increased reliance on the certainties in results. A further refinement was the belief that the greater the precision of measurement, the greater the validity of the findings. This, of course, is simply not true, or not necessarily true, because of prime importance is the validity of an application. In other words, a proposition may be entirely logical but it is not necessarily true.

The idea that a physical state can have profound effect upon an emotional or mental state is one side of the coin. The other is that a given mental or emotional state can influence the physical or physiological action of a drug. Both conditions are implicit in the widely used, and often misused, term *psychosomatic.*

STRESS

The *kind* of a physical symptom a person chooses, even if unconsciously, is often conditioned by the psychological factors in his background or in his make-up. While the concept is not necessarily new (the idea of target organs or organ inferiority having been previously described and often rejected), it is now looked upon with increasing open-mindedness. Clearly physical symptoms can be precipitated by stress if the stress has not been psychologically conditioned or adapted. In that case the behavioral or emotional safety valves cannot adequately handle the stress. The result is the appearance of physical symptoms, which may or may not be associated with organic causes. This suggests that physical symptoms due to demonstrated *organic* causes can be mediated—reduced or accentuated—by the psychological make-up of an individual. Although stress does not uniformly produce physical symptoms, physical disease often has stress as its origin.

If that is true, questions must arise on the reliability of our *well-controlled studies* in evaluating the effect of a drug. Man, the testing reagent, is the only uncontrolled variable in the test, by virtue of the variety of his ego defenses which are part of his psychological make-up.

Man naturally avoids stress. He attempts to attenuate the effect of stress by various methods, an important one being the ego defenses that he sets up to avoid facing an unpleasant event. An example thereof is denial, where a man does not wish to accept an apparent but unpleasant fact and thus saves himself from facing a stressful situation. Another example is the euphoria that patients with cancer or other diseases often develop. These defenses are useful indeed in such grave circumstances. Perhaps hope thus becomes a powerful ally in the remedial effect that a drug confers.

Measure of Stress: Stress or distress can produce clear physical signs. For example, both in physical stress and in depression, which is a psychological stress, there is a substantial increase in the secretion of 17-hydroxyketosteroids, one of the many hormones of the adrenal gland. Conversely, in an excited stage the secretion or level of 17-hydroxyketosteroids falls. Some influence that affects the fluctuation of 17-hydroxyketosteroids levels is the defense mechanism that man develops to handle his stress. That is one reason why the effect of a drug when studied in animals is not necessarily applicable to man, because as far as we know, animals have no psychological defense mechanisms. (Animals have other and simpler psychological reactions, such as avoidance behavior, but that cannot be equated with the powerful ego defenses that man has developed.) This is one situation where the evaluation of a drug in animals raises substantial questions as to comparability.

NERVOUS SYSTEM

These events are not surprising if we recall the simple fact that the function of the nervous system, which affects physiologically almost every function of the body, can be mediated by externally triggered events which affect thoughts and emotions. But we do not as readily accept the notion that the action of a drug can also be influenced by an emotional reaction or a thought. An example is an externally triggered event—as embarrassment, which is controlled by emotion or thought—that produces such a physiological happening as blushing.

DOCTOR–PATIENT

These are among the reasons why a doctor-patient relationship can be, under many circumstances, more critical than a drug-patient relationship. While a drug may adequately give a patient surcease, an understanding or perceptive physician may be vastly more helpful in the longer run. For example, people often fall apart due to a loss, whatever the loss may be. A person may adjust to the loss of a limb, difficult though it may be. But a loss of aspirations or loss of a treasured goal can be destructive to the psyche to the extent that the individual may not wish to undertake a recalibration of his aims and goals. He may rather give up when he loses his aims.

In the light of these events it appears inadequate to study the effect of a drug, even with most rigid double-blind controls, if the physician is blind to the breakdown in the patient's aspirations or self-acceptance. Death from grief due to a loss can thus, for example, become a fact rather than a dramatic expression.

ECOLOGY

Few actions or reactions are purely physical or purely psychological. A behavioral or emotional reaction such as aggression or hostility, while emotional in tone, is also strongly physiological or physical in mechanism, because hormonal factors play an integral role therein. We merely need to recall that castrated people, having lost sex glands that secrete hormones, are not commonly given to aggression.

Man does not function in separate compartments. His function is a totality of his physiological and psychological make-up. It would therefore appear that in an ecological sense, neither body nor mind specialists can afford to compete in the attempt to show which specialty is more important to man; but an integration of specialties should prove to be wholesome to him.

PHARMACOGENETICS

A variety of approaches and concepts in assessing drugs have had their ascendancy. Some were merely methodological, such as statistics and double-blind tests. Others were concepts, such as evaluations of predictability by study of the relationship between chemical structure and biological action. Now another old concept is demanding increasing attention, and it may considerably alter ideas in pharmacology. That concept is based on the fact that the genetic predisposition of an individual modifies the action of drugs he takes. This is the field of *pharmacogenetics,* an old phenomenon with a new name.

Not that genetic predisposition should be expected to solve all problems connected with the assessment of drugs. In fact, it poses problems or, rather, recognizes their existence. Pharmacogenetics merely recognizes or emphasizes that genetically determined conditions can modify the classical action of drugs in certain individuals, altering the metabolic conversion of these drugs or their degradation or their rate of excretion.

Thus pharmacogenetics can influence the effect and the toxicity of drugs.

GENETIC

Certain inborn conditions are known to make individuals more susceptible to the action of a given drug or more resistant to it. Errors of metabolism, basically heritable, genetically determined conditions, offer many examples, such as the crisis that can be precipitated by the administration of barbiturates in porphyria. Similarly, Roger Williams' thesis on the biochemical variability of individuals has emphasized that "normality" is variable due to variations in biological make-up. Williams considers the notion of the average or typical human being as an erroneous and a misleading one. (What we consider *normality* may merely be *frequency*.)

It is realized, too, that if the concept of pharmacogenetics were stretched to its extremity in its application to drug action, it would mean that no generalizations could be drawn. That extreme is not reflected by the facts; but on the other hand, the disregard of human variability—and differences in reaction to drugs due to that variability—cannot be ignored. We speak of individual variability; yet, in a larger scope, familial, ethnic or racial variability may be even more profound.

PHARMACOLOGICAL

Thus we cannot discuss the various types of metabolic conversions (detoxication mechanisms) without noting glaring exceptions. The proportion of such exceptions in the population is probably higher than we expect, due to multiple sensitivities. An individual who may have a sensitivity to a given drug may be sensitive to other drugs of the same family.

We speak glibly of the *action of drugs*. But such activity does not take place in a vacuum. There is not just the relationship of a drug to a metabolic state, but there is an interrelationship, due to the biological feedback mechanism, that is continuously taking place between a drug and metabolic products.

PHARMACOGENETICS

In this concern, it is easy to divide people into certain groups—as, for example, those who are taste responders to phenylthiourea and those who are not. To some people the taste of phenylthiourea—a chemical not used as a drug—is bitter; to others it is sweet. But such an oversimplification can grow into absurd classifications, as those who react to strawberries and those who do not. The field is more than classification; it is one that begs investigation.

The question also injects itself into other activity of drugs. What is applicable to or may be derived from one animal may not be applicable to others. For example, ACTH of sheep and cattle is identical; that of pig is different. This can be expected due to close phylogenetic relationship of sheep and cattle, but a departure from the pig. The difference is not the hormonally active portion of ACTH; but metabolism of the remaining part of the ACTH molecule may modify results, due to variability. Perhaps these responses should not be called "aberrant," but "different." The temptation is great to consider something atypical to be abnormal.

RAMIFICATIONS

Pharmacogenetic awareness highlights several problems. It emphasizes that transposition of data from *man to man* holds intrinsic questions of applicability. Certainly, the transposition of data from *animal to man* must be done with extreme forethought.

A second problem, dealing with the FDA views on safety and effectiveness, is one of more far-reaching effect. In interpreting its promulgated regulations, the FDA will probably bear in mind that the basis of many toxic reactions may be due to pharmacogenetic factors. Lay legislators to the contrary, occasional toxic reports should not invariably stigmatize a drug, for many a drug will exhibit a toxic reaction at some time in its career. This may not be due to its intrinsic toxicity but, like aspirin, primaquine, barbiturate, etc., due to individual intolerance. To create a fully antiseptic atmosphere for the public would logically demand the withdrawal of most drugs, including antibiotics, antimalarials, anesthetics, analgesics—all the way to zymogens. Each of them can precipitate a crisis when a reacting drug meets a susceptible individual.

Pharmacogenetics again focuses on the truism that the only invariable attribute of biological organisms is their variability.

BED REST

Illness is almost synonymous with bed rest. Even the expression *took to his bed* in English literature has for centuries meant to become ill. People, particularly neurotics, frequently go to bed or even lie down when the stresses become too much for them; the posture becomes one of illness, and illness is a respectable and accepted excuse for procrastination in dealing with responsibilities. To assume the horizontal position as a form of surrender is one thing; to assume that position for sleep is another. It is interesting to observe that when women take to bed as a result of an emotional upheaval, they usually lie on their face—prone. Whereas when either sex takes to bed as a result of exhaustion or to have a surcease from the stress of the world, they lie on their back—supine.

While bed rest in illness is a universal practice there is little to support the goodness of that universal remedy. Bed rest gives surcease and comfort but it also has side effects, some of which are damaging. We are speaking particularly of prolonged bed rest.

UNTOWARD EFFECTS

The horizontal position, prone or supine, causes a change in many organ positions. The adjustment to the new axis—a change in gravity—is often inimical to a patient. For example,

Browse,* who has investigated bed rest, states that "the heart works harder in the resting supine position than in resting erect." For that reason he wisely warns against indiscriminate bed rest, especially in those in whom the extra load on the heart may precipitate heart failure. Another untoward effect of bed rest, particularly after surgery, is thrombophlebitis, which possibly may herald death by a clot in the lung.

Prolonged bed rest has its particular dangers. Pneumonia, urinary infection, and kidney stones due to concentration of phosphates, calcium, and citrates may occur. Weakness or even wasting of muscles and calcium loss which leads to osteoporosis are some of its other dangers. There is, of course, a difference between short and prolonged bed rest, and untoward effects are usually negligible with the short bed rest of a few days. But even with a short bed rest, certain changes are apparent such as constipation. This may be due to a slowing of peristaltic motion or, more particularly, the new center of gravity may affect certain functions such as the ileogastric reflex.

The ileogastric reflex produces the urge to movement of stool immediately after a meal: a filled stomach sends a signal to the ileum to discharge its contents into the large intestine; if the pressure in the rectum is high enough, a discharge of stool takes place. This is actuated by nervous stimuli and takes place during an erect position—with its characteristic center of gravity—not during bed rest. That is one reason why people who are bedridden are likely to become constipated.

In coronary thrombosis, immobilization in bed is the customary procedure. Yet, bed rest increases the work of the heart. Bed rest may prove to be more tradition than treatment: the output of the heart is increased by 20% to 30% when lying down, about the same as in mild exercise. (There is a substantial difference, however, as exercise also increases heart *rate* but bed rest reduces it.)

In fact, the idea of bed rest is now being reexamined. A study was recently started on the virtues of getting around shortly after a heart attack.

* *The Physiology and Pathology of Bed Rest,* by N. L. Browse, Charles C Thomas, Springfield, Ill., 1965.

THE KILLER PAN

The bedpan is standard equipment to the bedridden. That, too, is a continuation of tradition. The process of using the bedpan to move bowels while in a lying position requires a bearing down, thus putting an intense strain on the heart. At times patients die on the bedpan from the effort. For this reason the use of a bedside commode, even for severely ill patients, is wisely more popular in many European countries.

There are other conditions in which chair rest, with feet hanging down, is more comfortable and safer than bed rest. One such condition is cardiac asthma. The circulatory load is eased by sitting in a chair. In fact, a change to a lying position in cardiac asthma, with a sudden influx into the vessels of blood which was in the legs, can precipitate heart failure and possibly death.

CHANGES

Many other changes of physiological function take place when lying down. There are also changes in kidney function. While the circulation in the kidneys is increased on short bed rest, the constitution of body fluids is changed upon prolonged bed rest. There are also a circulatory increase in muscles and peripheral vasodilation and an increase in the brain circulation upon lying down, a good empirical reason for placing a fainting person in a lying position.

WHEN DESIRABLE

Certain conditions do require bed rest—fracture, terminal illness, edema, varicose veins, or when there is another need of taking the weight off muscle or joint.

And perhaps for similar empirical reasons the horizontal state is used during diagnostic procedures. For example, there is a difference in electrocardiographic readings between sitting and lying, and the ECG is usually done with the patient lying. Yet it is perhaps more important to determine the potential of the heart during man's normal erect stance. Blood pressure reading will also differ between the upright and lying state, and even with a change in the position of the arm. Perhaps most physiological measurements should be made while the patient is erect and moving, his natural state, instead of lying down.

The events that take place during bed rest while awake are not the same as during sleep. During sleep there is a general slowing down and dampening of functions as respiration, urine secretion, bowel mobility, nervous reflex; but paradoxically there is a further increase in the blood flow in the brain.

PRONE–SUPINE

While precise information on bed rest is sparse indeed, there is less on the difference between the two horizontal positions—lying on one's back, *supine,* and lying on one's face, *prone.*

But there are at times sound psychological reasons that speak in favor of bed rest. The bed constitutes for some people a return to a safer and less demanding world. Therefore the physiological price may be well worth paying. The temporary surcease that the bed confers allows many people to return renewed to the stressful world in which they must live. For many, these changes in the function of the body take place if only to a negligible degree, during a short bed rest, as during a cold, fever, or stomach ache.

HICCUP

A hiccup is an arrested variant of breathing, a sudden and involuntary closure of the opening of the throat (glottis) during breathing. While occasionally it is considered funny—

though it is not—it is usually not serious. It is an interesting phenomenon due to the number of causes it may have. A hiccup may arise because of an irritating stimulus in the brain center that controls respiration and the function of the diaphragm, or such a stimulus in the nerve pathways themselves.

CAUSES

Few symptoms have as diverse an origin as hiccup. It may spring from disturbances resting in various organ systems; and in fact, in at least one condition, uremia, it may be a terminal sign. The diaphragm is always affected owing to its movement during hiccup. But the diaphragm may also be involved in the cause of hiccup, as when there is a hernia through the diaphragm or an abscess below it.

Hiccup may also be a symptom of an obstruction or an enlargement, irritating the nerve that is distributed through the diaphragm, the heart sac, and the pleurae. Hiccup may also be due to an intestinal or bronchial obstruction or tumor, a dilation of the stomach, or an enlargement of the heart. In an area as remote from the innervation of the phrenic nerve as the urinary bladder, irritation may occasionally produce hiccup. Hiccup may also be a sign of a neurological deficit or dysfunction. This is not surprising when the function of the brain in respiration is considered. And in senility, hiccup may accompany the degenerative changes that are associated with aging.

PSYCHOGENIC

Among the less serious origins of hiccup are hysteria and compulsive and uncontrollable laughter. This may occur in intensely reacting persons and may continue for days but cease during sleep. The hiccup of alcoholism is well known. It is probably due to irritation begun by toxic by-products of alcoholic metabolism, either by acetaldehyde or by the metabolic anomaly produced by the inactivation of an enzyme during an alcoholic bout. It disappears when the individual sobers up.

TREATMENT

The number of methods for treating hiccup is almost as varied as its causes. Stimulation of respiration through building up carbon dioxide by breathing with a paper bag over one's head is often successful. A favorite remedy of some decades ago was to frighten the patient by subjecting him to twists, turns, and somersaults in an airplane. Other measures still in use include pressure upon the eyeballs or upon the carotid artery, hyperventilation by breathing deeply and rapidly, the induction of nausea, or the conversion of a hiccup into a sneezing spell by tickling the nostrils with a feather.

Usually self-limiting and of no importance, hiccup often becomes a reason for merriment on the part of the onlookers, though the comedy therein is hard to fathom.

AGE OF ANXIETY

Tranquilizers are not the first agents used to influence a man's psyche. To alter the mental state people have been taking drugs for thousands of years, and for three basic purposes: to produce "liberation" or stupefaction, to derive exhilaration, or to develop hallucinations.

What does a people do for fun? The question is significant in that a people's amusements reflect their make-up, their values, and their philosophy. In fact, anthropologists frequently draw a profile of ethnic groups, ancient and modern, by studying how such groups divert themselves.

The majority of people in the world divert themselves through dancing, sex, and drugs. This is not extraordinary when one considers the population of many millions in the Near and Far East, and bears in mind that dancing is part of the religious rituals of many peoples. Social dancing is in vogue in every modern country.

LEISURE

Man's activity at work has a compelling component. Work imposes certain duties in its performance. Man's personality is not necessarily reflected in his work—owing to the obligation of doing what has been prescribed for the job or in performing what the job demands. When man does not have the compulsion to do, or the prohibition against doing, certain acts, he can give free rein to doing what he likes. And in doing what he likes, he reflects his inner self.

CARRYOVER

However, work is frequently so demanding or the competitive pressures during work are so stressful that man's fun and leisure often become merely an emotional extension of his work. He works at his play. An example thereof is the habit of talking shop at social gatherings to the extent that one's business often becomes one's sole preoccupation. By and large, this condition applies to our contemporary scene. For example, the notion "I-work-hard-and-play-hard" has social approbation and unfortunately carries a cachet of social acceptance.

This set of circumstances creates tensions, and therewith a need of reducing the tension that carries over into activities after the day's work. Many find that alcohol reduces the wrought-up pitch. Others find that sedatives will sandbag the excitement developed during the day but which continues through the evening. For some, tranquilizers offer a respite without the cerebral dulling that accompanies sedatives.

DRUGS

The term *drug* conjures up a bad connotation. By some, drug and dope are considered to be synonyms. But at all times and in all cultures drugs have been prominent in the social life of a people. They were used to liberate them by creating a forgetfulness (opium or alcohol), to exhilarate them (hashish), or to produce hallucinations (mescal buttons or hallucinogenic mushrooms). Some drugs, such as hashish, were used for both exhilaration and hallucination by creating alterations in time, depth and color perception. All of these drugs created social, as well as individual, problems.

The use of drugs politically or as war matériel is not strange. The Japanese distributed opium to make people more tractable to their political ambitions. The white settlers in America used alcohol, among other matériel, to win the country from the Indians. Agent provocateurs provided alcohol to the Indians to stir them up, so that a respectable excuse was at hand to put them down. While an Indian would not disclose war plans under torture, he would betray them while drunk with alcohol, for which he had an extremely low threshold. Measles and alcohol probably carried off more Indians than gunpowder.

With the long, and at times infamous, history of drugs, it is strange to find a squeamishness or mock righteousness that considers the supervised use of drugs antisocial. It is stranger yet to find that in the same breath the use of one particular drug, alcohol, is extolled by social approbation.

It is extraordinary to find that the thoughtful and professionally supervised uses of tranquilizers are scored as the instruments for brainwashing, as devices that reduce the competitive spirit and breed a state of complacency, or as addicting, habit-forming substitutes for dope.

Is it possible that our Puritanical spirit is stronger than scientific objectivity?

TRANQUILIZERS

The remedy that is good for all ills is good for no ill. By the same token, antibiotics are not the treatment for every infection, and a real danger exists in their use when an antibiotic takes the place of diagnosis.

Similarly, tranquilizers are not a substitute for assessing behavioral problems, correcting or adjusting to environmental stresses, or taking an inventory of an emotional make-up. As with antibiotics, they are not a substitute for diagnosis.

Tranquilizers have reduced the population of mental institutions. They have placed those emotionally ill into a frame of mind so that they are more amenable, reachable, for treatment by a psychiatrist. But the greatest good, in numbers alone, is rendered to the anxious and competitive man, who will be more effective when his hostility, defensiveness and overanxiety are tempered, under medical supervision, by the judicious use of tranquilizers.

Competition for economic survival takes a most illogical turn when it is concluded that the elimination of anxiety removes the competitive spirit. Thus anxiety is made a virtue, and stress a sign of competence. It is an age of anomaly indeed if it fears to relax; relaxation revivifies, refills, and refreshes and allows man to rise to greater accomplishment.

This does not mean that tranquilizers should become supplements to the daily vitamin intake. Neither does it mean that tranquilizers should be used instead of solving a problem, for they may be subjected to the same abuse that alcohol is put to. But it does mean that to deplore their use as killers of initiative is absurd.

Society keys up the individual to strive in his competitive endeavor. It should not cast a social frown upon drugs that can replenish his reserves. It is absurd to deplore mental illness resulting from stress or somatic conditions such as hypertension, to which emotional stress is a contributing factor, and then deplore the supervised use of relatively safe drugs which may reduce illness-provoking stress, obviously, under thoughtful, professional advice. We must not forget that over two centuries ago, coffee was considered a dangerous drug and was controlled by legislation.

BIOCHEMISTRY AND THE MENTAL STATE

There seems to be no shame in admitting to a bellyache or any other "physical" disease. But the word "mental" still triggers a strong reaction in the mind of the ordinary individual when applied to him or to a relative. Any disturbance that has to do with the mental function, or an emotional condition, is still fraught with shame, or guilt, or defenses. This is despite the canon that the body and mind are not separate entities.

Regrettably, disputes also range among investigators in the mental and emotional areas, and they are more than mere differences of opinion. These disputes are predominantly between two antipodal philosophies: (a) that mental and emotional disturbances are due to environmental stresses and can be treated by psychotherapy, i.e., psychoanalysis and other verbal analytic methods which attempt to ferret out and interpret early environmental aspects which may be precursors of the present anomalous behavior, and (b) that mental and emotional disturbances are due to metabolic or biochemical defects which interfere with sound behavior and can be treated by chemotherapy.

The acerbity of the disputes creates confusion; and perhaps the old aphorism applies, that *truth more likely can spring from error than from confusion.* The fact may well be—and it so appears by many signs—that there is no unitary cause, but that the origin of mental and emotional disturbances resides in the psychological, pharmacological, and physiological, including the genetic areas.

CLASSIFICATION

Occasionally people do become involved in classification as an end in itself. Verbal ballistics is the joy of pedants. Nevertheless there are a great many reasons for the need for classification of diseases. There is a need to apply *labels* at least for one reason, among others: the label fixes what we mean by a term, enables us to convey a concept, and helps assure that with the use of the label, which is merely a symbol, there is common consensus on what we mean by it.

Confusion in psychiatry has been partially due to a diversity of nomenclature. The American Psychiatric Association has considerably helped to reduce nomenclatural confusion by the publication of its *Manual of Mental Disorders.* Even that requires revisions, but above all, it requires common and universal use.

WHAT TO CALL IT

One thing that contributes to the substantial problem in classification is the question of nomenclature. How should mental and emotional disturbances be named? By causes? These are usually unknown. By symptoms? The same or similar symptoms often characterize different conditions. By prognosis? Usually not predictable. By defects or failures of function? That would be often merely descriptive, as, for example, the term *hypersplenism* merely means enlarged spleen but says nothing of origin, pathology, prognosis; and hypersplenism may be associated with a number of quite unrelated conditions.

DYNAMIC METHODS

The methods referred to as *dynamic, analytic,* or *psychoanalytic* are attempts to approach by verbal means the understanding or treatment of disturbances of emotional functions. The patient expresses himself to the psychotherapist who often goes back to his early childhood, evaluates, and relates the patient's story to the problems for which the patient now seeks help.

There are many schools of thought and methods in the dynamic method. Some interpret and advise the patient (directive therapy) ; others use a so-called nondirective method, sitting more or less passively and listening, based on the idea that the patient will gain insight into his problems and resolve them himself. Both proponents and opponents, vigorously and at times vituperatively, espouse their adherence or dissent. The opponents point to the lack of strict controls; the proponents point out the empirical successes. Opponents' rebuttal says that a given percentage get well anyway. Proponents' rejoinder says that patients did not get well, for which reason they sought help. The simple fact is that we are not at a stage where capsules can aid an individual to gain insight, develop judgment, or handle his characterological problems. Despite the schisms and skews, sexual problems such as impotence, frigidity, and mental vaginismus cannot be handled by drugs, and they may spread stress in other areas of an individual's behavior.

Because of the acceptance of analysis on the part of many public figures and its engendered vogue, emotional and mental anomalies are becoming somewhat less fraught with feelings of shame, guilt, and prudishness than heretofore. The dynamic methods have thus been a powerful factor in creating public interest in mental health.

BIOLOGICAL METHOD

Often referred to as *biological psychiatry* or the *psychopharmacological* approach to the study, diagnosis and treatment of mental and emotional disturbances, this method rests on the belief that there is a metabolic or biological cause for these disturbances. But within the biological schools of thought there are a variety of hypotheses or theories. They attempt to unearth what accounts for biochemical defect, mental and emotional disturbances.

In the biological field some schools of thought direct their attention to schizophrenia; others to depression or disturbances of other affects, degenerative diseases such as senile cerebral arteriosclerosis or the chronic brain syndrome, or anxiety reactions including panic. The attention to schizophrenia is perhaps the most widespread. But biological psychiatrists cannot handle such problems as strengthening defenses such as denial in anticipated death, nor failure of adaptive behavior in ministering to a marriage falling apart, nor intellectualizing on the part of patients as a form of rationalization. Nor can they treat denial when it is a defense to be removed to prevent repression, which is its internal counterpart. Denial is the external one. But dynamic or analytical psychiatrists do treat these problems, which may be petty but have overwhelming consequences. Perhaps it requires merely a knowledgeable individual with insight instead of an analyst. Nonetheless, in these situations, the dynamic practitioner is the recourse for the patient.

Biological psychiatrists react strongly to the label *dynamic*. The dynamic practitioners react strongly to a variety of labels. With some, their brand of analysis is not a science or an art but an ideology which is belabored with zeal and exhibitions of antipathy to anything other than the brand dispensed by them. It becomes a priesthood with its rituals and dogmas, and when that occurs there is an unintentional exploitation of the person seeking help.

SCHIZOPHRENIA

Schizophrenia is frequently a severe and profound personality disorganization, often described as splitting or dissociation of a personality. This refers to situations in which the so-called *normal* reaction is dissociated or split into its affective (emotional) and ideational (thinking) forms, as when the emotional meaning is taken out of the context of a happening. A good example is a funeral wherein the happening is a burial. The normal reaction in our culture is sadness, the emotional component of the happening. A schizophrenic person may laugh, divorcing the emotional meaning from the actual happening. This is an inappropriate reaction; in fact, inappropriate reactions, in part, characterize schizophrenia.

Biological psychiatrists believe the cause to be chemical, perhaps triggered in genetic soil. Dynamic adherents believe the cause to be environmental—societal and familial. And among the biological schools there is a difference of opinion on the nature and cause of the metabolic defect that leads to the perceptual anomaly that schizophrenia presents. Among ideas proposed, each with reasonable evidence, are (a) there is a defect in carbohydrate utilization; (b) there are disturbances in the energy cycle wherein a biochemical reaction, oxidative phosphorylation, is disturbed; (c) there are anomalies in amino acid metabolism, with evidence partially adduced by the mental disturbances that are associated with errors of metabolism like phenylketonuria; (d) in the catecholamine (epinephrine) hypothesis, oxidation products of epinephrine (adrenaline) are said to produce adrenochrome and adrenolutin acting as psychotogens, for which the use of nicotinic acid has been reported to be considerably helpful; (e) the ceruloplasmin hypothesis is also related to epinephrine oxidation. Adrenochrome, a metabolite or oxidation product of epinephrine, is also found in normals, but in schizophrenics it is found in very much larger amounts. There are differences of opinion on the role of adrenochrome, and another factor enters: in the psychotic or schizophrenialike state that occurs by administration of LSD, there is also increased adrenochrome excretion. Interpretation appears easier than it is.

It is difficult to treat schizophrenia. But it is also difficult to characterize schizophrenia with precision. Recognized by its symptoms of personality disorganization, often with hallucination, paranoid ideas with depersonalization, thought unrelatedness and inappropriateness, it is probably not a disease *per se,* but a cluster of diseases, or reactions, producing a change in personality. Man reacts with stress to a precarious or untenable situation; schizophrenia may be, in part, a reaction to an untenable or intolerable situation, partially environmental, which, overlaid on a genetically fertile soil, may produce metabolic changes through which schizophrenia is precipitated. This is not inconsistent with the hypothesis of biological psychiatry; stress produces metabolic alterations in bodily functions. The psyche and soma are not separate entities. Emotions, producing stress, affect the nervous system and particularly the endocrinological system including functions of the thyroid and the adrenals, the latter secreting epinephrine among other hormones or hormonelike substances. The induction of faulty metabolic handling by the body of epinephrine—the basis of one hypothesis—is not an unwarranted leap. But again, schizophrenia may not be a single metabolic disease.

The matter of cause of schizophrenia is complicated by additional factors. It has a variety of sensory disturbances, which may be either cause or effect or neither, for they may be merely associated with it. Sensory disturbances can be produced by *clearly environmental* conditions, as by sensory deprivation. An example of such stress is evident in monkeys raised without mothers or mother substitutes.

RESEARCH PROBLEMS

The research problems in biological aspects of psychiatry are considerable. For example, there is a lack of a reliable model of schizophrenia on which research can be based. Here, too, we have a situation that is bizarre. On the one hand, we have no adequate or valid model, but on the other, some hold that amphetamine or LSD often produces a syndrome indistinguishable from schizophrenia. Can the model be considered to be a replica of a disease when the disease has such varied manifestations? Another difficulty resides in proof. We are looking for *conclusive* proof, and in the search we may be discarding evidence which, while not conclusive, may lead to it. In a condition such as schizophrenia, which takes many forms, the rigid requirement of the scientific method may not be scientific at all, or even sensical.

Ordinarily, compounds carry certain inherent toxicities. Yet, compounds that are not ordinarily toxic may become toxic to schizophrenics—the pattern of errors of metabolism. However, almost every finding reported has been countermanded by negative results by other researchers.

Commonly, urine and blood serum of schizophrenics are used in studies of drug excretion or in the search for metabolites uniquely present in schizophrenics. But in a disordered metabolism that is basic, patterns cannot be expected, so reliance on other common research measures is reduced. For example, the urinary excretion of norephinephrine is decreased in some cases of depression and is increased in others. Such variation in excretion studies also occurs with hormones, electrolytes, and some proteins. Recently, the "pink spots" finding in the urine of schizophrenics has been reported to occur in urine of nonschizophrenics as well. Biological cycles will also give a variance in observed results; a drug administered in the morning may not give the same end-products when administered at night.

In any work, one must start with certain assumptions. But the assumption that a toxic substance shown to be present in blood or urine (or a normal substance absent) may be only a half truth, for the presence of the toxic substance may require additional conditions for it to exert its toxic effect.

There is promise in the luxuriantly increasing investigations of sleep and dreams. This is not, as heretofore, limited to the dynamic schools. For example REM sleep has been found to be increased by LSD; barbiturates, alcohol, and particularly amphetamine have been reported to suppress REM sleep. (REM sleep is the early part of a sleep cycle characterized by dreams, and during which there are *r*apid *e*ye *m*ovements.)

DRUGS

Aside from the sedatives and now commonplace tranquilizers, a number of drugs are used in the treatment of mental and emotional diseases. Some drugs were used predominantly as research tools, such as LSD.

A considerable number of drugs are concerned with the monoamines of the brain. The most important are norepinephrine and dopamine (catecholamines) and serotonin (an indole amine). A deficiency of serotonin is believed to be involved in schizophrenia and in depression.

Among antidepressants, monoamine oxidase (MAO) inhibitors and imipramine are the principal drugs used. They lift the mood in depression, probably by increasing the amount of circulating norepinephrine in the brain. MAO inhibitors, *inhibit the inhibitor,* i.e., the oxidase that deactivates monoamines. The objective is to raise the level of monoamines in the brain. Reserpine lowers norepinephrine and serotonin in the brain, which is the principal reason for its depressing effect.

The use of nicotinic acid or niacinamide is based on its

supposedly deactivating effect on adrenochrome as a psychotogen. Whether that is the mechanism of action is not broadly accepted, but the reports on the effect of nicotinic acid are encouraging.

Many important drugs are not mentioned here. Among them are drugs used as research tools as well as in treatment, e.g., acetylcholine, controlling the firing of the "spark plugs of the brain," and others. This discussion, touching only the peaks, is perforce much oversimplified.

SYNCRETISM

Progress in the mental area was essentially slow due to the dearth of conceptual thinking as well as methodology up to quite recently. In view of the complexity and the wide areas of ignorance, none can afford to be dogmatic. *The enemy is mental and emotional disturbances—not a researcher in another discipline.* It would appear that clarification and understanding will probably arise from *both* the dynamic and biological schools of thought. Personal vendettas may salve little egos but they do not solve problems.

CLOCKS AND RHYTHMS IN LIVING ORGANISMS

We are familiar with the rhythm of the heartbeat, an action composed of two different events which recur in man, at rest, about 70 times a minute. The rhythm differs in other animals —about 35 times per minute in the horse, about 1000 times in the canary, and probably close to 2000 times in the hummingbird. Even the *components* of the heartbeat have their own rhythm which is timed to the split second—in man, 0.3 second for contraction (systole) of the ventricles and 0.5 second for their relaxation (diastole). It is this order that enables the heart to rest for about 20 years during a lifetime, in the form of rest periods of less than a second between each beat.

CYCLES

A recurring event or a cycle presupposes a regularity—a predictable, fixed interval after which recurrence takes place. This is responsive to a built-in biological clock. There are various lengths of a cycle, and the timing varies among different functions, but it is always the same in a given function. For example, in man there is a sleep cycle, recurring every 24 hours; menstrual cycle recurring about every 28 days; the previously mentioned heartbeat recurring about 70 times a minute; and the learned habits, such as feeding and excretion, which recur regularly.

Cycles are often related to the day-night sequence. Man's is the day cycle of activity. Mice and other nocturnal animals have a night cycle of activity. The tides, the night and day sequence, the moon, the seasons of the year, etc., all follow a specific cycle: occurrence, cessation, and recurrence. In fact, because such events recur they facilitate study such as comparison and determination of what other events influence them.

PHYSIOLOGICAL EVENTS

Most physiological events in man follow a certain periodic pattern. For example, the adrenal gland has a circadian (about 24 hours) rhythm, increasing the elaboration of its hormones during sleep. They are at their height early in the day as a stimulant to activity. Their secretion declines as the day advances. They have performed one of their activities—as a starter.

This phenomenon is related to and can be used to enhance the activity of a drug, depending on what part of the day it is administered. For example, the responsiveness to ACTH is greater at the end of the day, when the natural function of the adrenal is low, than in the morning when it is high. Resistance also alters with the cycle. Mice can withstand inoculation with *E. coli* endotoxin reasonably well when given at the height of their cycle, which is at midnight, but more often they succumb when it is injected at noon, their low. This is the pattern of nocturnal animals.

The occurrence of wide swings from regularity may herald disease—as, for example, low blood sugar or hypoglycemia, which often signals the onset of diabetes. Other internal timing mechanisms, often related to light or darkness as with birds or insects, control certain other physiological functions or behavioral effects. Light-darkness cycles can be disturbed by holding an animal for 24-hour periods in light or in darkness. These timing devices or functions are not limited to large animals but occur even in single-celled organisms.

DISTURBANCE OF CYCLES

It follows that disturbances of natural cycles have their grave results, physiologically and psychologically. Passengers who traverse several time zones often develop temporary but often moderate to severe discomforts which prevent them from functioning at their usual competence, pace, and comfort. The problem is much multiplied in jet pilots making lateral runs across several time zones, for unlike passengers who travel occasionally, pilots traverse the time zones frequently. The disturbance of their biological rhythm often produces wide fluctuation in weight, tension and fatigue, impotence or disturbances of sleep, and changes in emotional stability. The need to adapt to a different metabolic pattern in connection with eating and other habits, only to change the adaptation rapidly, may be one of the causes for such disturbances in pilots. The same problems are encountered by people who experiment with 6- to 12-hour cycles compared with the normal 24-hour cycle in daily living, or who draw their drapes and remain secluded without awareness of the day-night sequence.

The principle of disorganizing the biological clock can be compared to upsetting the timing on an electric clock-thermostat which controls an oil burner. This apparatus makes two complete clock revolutions in one 24-hour period. When changing the clock from daylight to standard time by moving the hands ahead 11 hours, the apparatus will be upset. It will follow the night cycle of reduced heat during the day, and conversely, will give off more heat, following the day cycle, during the night. If the clock hands are moved ahead 23 hours or moved back one hour, no disturbance in its preset mechanism will occur.

Since the function of biological clocks and time mechanisms in living organisms is fundamental, it was astounding to read a story in a New York newspaper which labeled an account of the biological clock in roaches (which respond to the day-night sequence) as a *most spectacular scientific nonsequitur of many a day*. That condescending and uninformed opinion was given despite the report that in implanting two different biological clocks in roaches they developed tumors which were believed to be intestinal cancer!

HYPNOSIS

Hypnosis is a state of somnolence, not necessarily sleep, which can be induced in an individual. During that stage his suggestibility is immensely increased, and he can act upon the suggestion given him during this time. The phenomenon of hypnosis or suggestion therapy during a trance has been used for centuries in the treatment of disease. Suggestion therapy has played a key role in Egypt—note the physician-priests. In pastoral counseling today suggestion also plays a strong part. Successful hypnosis requires that the person hypnotized accept wholly and uncritically the suggestions of the hypnotist or operator.

Aside from the use of hypnosis for entertainment, which must be clearly and unquestionably condemned, its current greatest usefulness is in therapy, usually by trained and experienced physicians or by other skilled and responsible hypnotists.

MYTHS

There are certain myths about hypnosis. People categorically fear uncritical acceptance as dangerous, but an uncritical acceptance of suggestions by the hypnotist is imperative. While uncritical acceptance may indeed expose one to deceit and demagoguery, much depends upon the setting in which such uncritical acceptance takes place. *In fact when we learn something new we must first uncritically accept its teaching until we know enough about the subject to enable us to look upon it critically.*

For example, everyone has uncritically accepted the multiplication table. In hypnosis, there must be uncritical acceptance by the subject or patient of the operator's directions, instructions, and suggestions for the hypnotic event to be successful. The hypnotist persuades in the induction of the hypnotic state, and then orders in giving the suggestion. Both must be wholly accepted. Resistance on the part of the patient precludes successful hypnosis.

Another myth is that only "weak minds" can be hypnotized. The fact is that it requires a reasonable amount of intelligence to be put under a hypnotic trance, as the subject must have the ability to concentrate. He must also understand enough to be able to accept an idea, which an idiot may not be able to do. And the patient must be intelligent enough to have a motivation to participate in the hypnotic event.

Another of the many myths is that only persons with "weak wills" can be hypnotized, and therefore some rigidly resist the directions of the hypnotist, to demonstrate the strength of their will. But rigidity is frequently an overcompensation for uncertainty rather than evidence of strength. A good parallel is stubbornness, which is the strength of the weak.

INDUCTION

Physiologically and emotionally man responds to a variety of stimuli: (1) chemical, on the basis of which psychoactive drugs such as antidepressants are used; (2) electrical, through impulses or stimuli sent by implanted electrodes; (3) signals that may be verbal, visual, or auditory.

A state of hypnosis can be induced by verbal signals, such as by monotonous and repetitive suggestions. It can be aided by objects, such as a spot on the wall or other stationary or moving objects to which the hypnotist directs the attention of the subject. It can be induced by person-to-person contact between hypnotist and subject or by remote means, as by television.

The principle, however, by whatever method hypnosis is induced, is the concentration or attention of the subject to the directions and suggestions of the hypnotist. A hypnosislike state can be induced by a public address. Political demagogues like Hitler and Castro are examples. The state so induced is mass hypnosis, wherein a mob is sent into a hypnoidal state. Surely, here, critical appraisal of what the speaker is saying would preclude a hypnoidal state.

The hypnotic trance is somewhere between the waking and sleeping states. While five stages of increasing depth of trance are recognized, comparatively little is known of the nature of hypnosis. There is probably more definite and reproducible knowledge about sleep than about hypnosis.

We know hypnosis by its effects: a stage of suggestibility during which profound relaxation of muscle takes place but not relaxation of sphincters and there is a reduction of stress, both physical and psychic. The subject may appear to be asleep but is usually easily aroused, and paradoxically he may be in a deep trance but can open his eyes on command.

THE HYPNOTIST

The person of the hypnotist is a weighty factor in the induction of the hypnotic state. The hypnotist may be a physician if hypnosis is used in the treatment of disease or in psychiatric states, or he may be an experienced hypnotist when the purpose of treatment is to change delinquent habit states, such as poor study habits in students, a desire to overeat, etc. Or he may be a dentist when the objective of the hypnotic state is to create partial anesthesia or analgesia in dental treatment. Hypnosis is used by physicians in the treatment of diseases of various systems, but particularly by psychiatrists in emotional disturbances.

Much is made of the person of the hypnotist. Some believe that he carries the seeds of grandiosity and a fantasy for omnipotent power in his control over his subject. Perhaps Lord Acton's statement, "Power corrupts—absolute power corrupts absolutely," can apply here too.

MANIPULATION

Due to the power held by the hypnotist, there is a distinct danger in his manipulation of the patient or subject. In fact, the reverse may also apply, as a patient can learn how to manipulate the hypnotist. But power plays are a normal component of interaction among people, and it is merely that in a hypnotic setting the likelihood may be greater. However, awareness of the danger reduces its own problem, which is probably limited to only occasional individual encounters.

A person can manipulate the hypnotist by feigning to be in a hypnotic trance or by other actions. Incidentally, there is no certain method to determine whether a subject is truly in a hypnotic trance or not. He may easily learn to feign, dissemble, and simulate. While this does not serve him constructively, the mere act of manipulation may give the patient satisfaction.

It is held that a subject will reject any suggestion by the hypnotist which may be against his principles or notions of morality. But different opinions on this point also exist. Though in a different setting, political brainwashing works, and that too is persuasion and suggestion which may originally have been against the principles of the subject.

THERAPY

A variety of conditions are successfully treated by hypnosis. The earliest condition treated was pain in attempts to produce anesthesia and analgesia in surgery. Pain is still perhaps the most widely treated condition, including pain of cancer. Other conditions treated are gastrointestinal disturbances, neuralgia, asthma, vomiting of pregnancy, hypertension, Raynaud's phenomenon (which is a blanching of fingers and toes due to local inhibition of circulation), and even, though not surprisingly, dermatological conditions. Since relaxation is reduction of stress, it is clear that the diseases of stress such as high blood pressure should be ameliorated by hypnosis, which relaxes. (Hypnosis may also be used to produce great rigidity of muscle.)

DANGERS

As with almost any measure, there is a danger associated with hypnosis if it is misused or misapplied, due perhaps to its striking, almost magical nature. But there is little danger that a patient will be put into a trance and will not be able to be aroused. Even if the hypnotist forgets the signal he gave the patient for arousal, a hypnotic trance is self-limited and the subject will awaken spontaneously, but perhaps many hours later.

However, the greatest danger in hypnosis lies in the removal of symptoms and defenses. Pain may be a symptom of a deep-seated condition which needs treatment. If the pain is removed a false security may be engendered; the condition remains while the symptoms, i.e., pain, disappears.

And the removal of defenses may cause a psychiatric problem. Defenses are substitutes that many people use; the example of overeating to overcome loneliness or lack of acceptance by peers is well known. When a defense is removed, another more harmful defense may be substituted by the patient. An example of a substitution of a worse defense is addiction to drugs or alcoholism for overeating.

A defense is often the only guard an individual may have to protect himself from what may appear an assailment to his own ego. The fact that no defense is necessary does not occur to him. Or he may not trust himself without a defense for a fearful but imaginary danger. At times a physical symptom is a person's defense.

Thoughtless removal of such a defense may precipitate depression. Removal of a defense, without adequate treatment of the underlying condition or without substituting a milder defense may even, in rare cases, precipitate suicide which can follow depression.

There is nothing magical about the extraordinary feats that are reported to take place during a hypnotic trance. They are evidence of man's potential, of his powers when he is not blocking or otherwise limiting himself. Other feats that appear extraordinary appear to be so merely because one is not normally called upon to perform them: a common one enables a person to remain lying straight when supported only by his heels and the back of his head. This is accomplished by muscle rigidity induced hypnotically.

Hypnosis, as a method of treatment in expert hands, is effective and relatively safe in certain well-considered conditions. But it is not an instant cure nor instant psychiatry, nor does it serve as a magic wand.

ENZYMES

Not long ago, the public became quite well acquainted with enzymes in connection with detergents. However, enzymes have been long with us. In fact, man continues to live because enzymes enable a variety of numerous functions to take place in the human body.

Enzymes used in medicine and commonly known are pepsin, papain, and pancreatin. These are involved in digestion. They represent only a small portion of the number of enzymes elaborated by the human organism. There are numerous other enzymes in medicine for various purposes. In industry, enzymes play a determining role: certain materials such as textiles, paper, and leather can be made better through enzyme technology. The sheer existence of these industries is made possible by enzyme technology: the distilling, brewing, and dairy industries producing wine, beer, and cheese owe their existence to enzymes.

A proteolytic enzyme is one that digests protein. An amylolytic enzyme is one that digests starches or carbohydrates. A cellulolytic enzyme is one that digests cellulose.

Enzymes are organic materials elaborated by living tissue, acting as catalysts accelerating biochemical reactions. They are characterized by many qualities, but enzymes are specific and exclusive in their action, which is a broad statement regarding biological mechanisms. In other words, a given enzyme will have only one effect and will act only on a specific substance creating a specific end product. Enzymes function at their best at certain temperatures, at certain narrow limits of acidity, and on specific substances called substrates.

Enzymes act upon a substrate and convert the material on which they act, the substrate, into end products. More specifically, milk diastase, which is an enzyme acting upon carbohydrates, converts its substrate, starch, into maltose.

ANTIENZYMES

But enzymes can easily be destroyed, by antienzymes. The best known antienzyme is heat; most enzymes are killed above 40° C (104° F), and all of them are killed by boiling. In fact, the velocity of enzyme action is accelerated with increasing temperature until 35° C to 40° C, after which the activity decreases and eventually the enzyme is killed. The preservation of certain foods by boiling is an example of the use of heat as an antienzyme, for heat kills the enzyme that causes the foodstuff to deteriorate. Many antiseptics are antienzymes when they inhibit enzyme action. If the inhibition is irreversible, the enzyme is killed. Enzymes can also be inhibited by a degree of acidity which is not the optimum for the activity of that particular enzyme. Thus a substantial change in degree of acidity acts as an antienzyme. A change in degree of acidity does not necessarily destroy an enzyme, but it prevents it from functioning.

Though enzymes are specific and exclusive in their activity, as a given enzyme will convert only a given, specific substance, antienzymes are not as specific or exclusive. For example, heat which acts as an antienzyme will inactivate or kill *any* enzyme. By and large, however, antienzymes also have specific properties in inhibiting specific enzymes.

A good example of a substance with antienzyme activity is sodium lauryl sulfate, a detergent.

ENZYMES IN MEDICINE

Much has been done in the use of enzymes in therapy since Berzelius postulated the existence of enzymes in 1830 and since Kuhne in 1867 proposed the term *enzyme* to describe the organic catalysts elaborated by living matter which accelerate a biochemical reaction. The advances in the biochemistry of enzymes, which includes their identification and their physical chemistry, their mechanism of action, and finally the crystallization of a number of enzymes, added to our knowledge concerning them.

Enzymes have been employed as physiological tools in research as well as in diagnosis. Their physiological properties have been studied and their role in health and disease investigated. Many of the studies have attempted to answer basic questions, such as the reason why pepsin, which digests protein, does not digest the stomach itself, which secretes it. The reason for this unusual phenomenon is *believed* to be an antienzyme to pepsin which prevents its digestion of the stomach. That explanation, however, has not been experimentally demonstrated. But it has been established that enzymes digest cells that have been killed, not living cells. Nevertheless, the pitcher plant may be an exception to that rule, for it is believed to digest the insects it entraps. There is also a theory contradictory thereto which holds that the plant digests the insect after it has died.

ENZYMES IN THERAPY

Based on the premise that enzymes will digest dead cells, a number of enzymes are used for cleaning up dead tissue in wounds. Trypsin, a proteolytic enzyme secreted by the pancreas, is applied to dead tissue in order to hasten its dissolution. Streptokinase-streptodornase, which are enzymes elaborated by hemolytic streptococci, are also used for that purpose.

Hyaluronidase, an enzyme broadly distributed in the animal world, increases tissue permeability. For that reason hyaluronidase has been called a *spreading factor.* It has been employed to aid the spread of injected solutions such as local anesthetics or antibiotics, or to prevent the accumulation of solid matter which results in kidney stones. Its experimental use has been described in a variety of other conditions. An enzyme from muscle, adenosine-5-monophosphoric acid or its sodium salt, has been reported to be useful in a number of conditions, which include collagen and skin diseases, and new uses for it are regularly reported.

A chemical substance, acetazolamide, has recently been found to function as an antienzyme and has been used as a diuretic. Acetazolamide inhibits carbonic anhydrase, one of the enzymes involved in the filtration of urine, and thus by diuresis it (acetazolamide) stimulates water and salt excretion. Quite the opposite effect–i.e., inhibition of excretion in order to retain penicillin–is accomplished by another chemical, carinamide, which has in this instance also the function of an antienzyme.

OTHER ENZYMES

It has been said that all of physiology is fundamentally a study of enzymes and multienzyme systems. Perhaps that is an oversimplified view, though enzymes appear to have a fundamental bearing in almost every biochemical mechanism. At least coenzymes or enzyme precursors play a role in almost every vital physiological function. These functions are fundamental because they underlie the gross appearance of a physiological function. For example, the process of human respiration is well known; underlying that are the processes of respiration of the cells, which are triggered by the respiratory enzymes. Respiration has been defined as the sum total of the processes that introduce oxygen into the system and remove carbon dioxide. A number of respiratory enzymes, oxygenases and dehydrogenases, are therein concerned. Cytochrome C, broadly speaking, is one such enzyme: when in an oxidized form it gives off its oxygen in cell metabolism and is thereby reduced, only to be again oxidized, and the cell accepts the oxygen it carries and is thereby again reduced in the unique and fantastically functioning organization which is the continuous process of cell respiration.

OBESITY OR OVERWEIGHT

DEFINITION

Obesity is an increase of body weight, predominantly fat, usually 10% or more above what a "normal" weight is considered to be according to the standard height-frame-weight tables. Obesity is always overweight, though overweight is not necessarily obesity. Overweight is an increase of 10% or more of body weight (not necessarily fat) over that considered to be the normal weight by these tables. While overweight and obesity are not necessarily synonyms, they can well be considered to be the same for practical purposes.

Hunger is a painful or at least an uncomfortable sensation in the stomach. It occurs usually when the stomach is empty. Hunger is accompanied by peristaltic waves in the stomach walls, felt as or accompanied by pangs ("hunger pangs") or a hollow feeling, crying to be filled. It is relieved by food intake—though not invariably, as will be discussed later.

Appetite is something else; it is a pleasant anticipatory feeling characterized by a desire for the pleasant sensation of eating.

CAUSE

There is one simple cause for obesity: the consumption of more food than is necessary for outgoing energy expenditure.

This applies even in the rare occasion when obesity is due to a "glandular" condition or due to a genetic predisposition. In those conditions too, the energy expenditure is also less than the food intake. Either energy expenditure is too low or food intake is too high. There may be a number of reasons why certain persons have a smaller output of energy, not balanced with the intake of food.

DISCUSSION AND CAUTIONS

It is often a mistake to urge people to reduce. Fat serves a purpose. The process of acquiring it is associated with the comfort of eating—usually too well. Food has a sedative action; the relaxation and unwinding after having dined or supped are traditional. Fat or obesity is also a buffer. Metaphorically, it protects the fat person from the outside world—warding off anxiety, exorcising the devils figuratively that literally do not exist. But even if they exist only symbolically or figuratively, they appear real!

Food is a comfort, an anxiety-reducing measure due to its sedative or relaxing value. The greater the anxiety the greater or more frequent will be the intake of food, in the search for equanimity, peace, relaxation, or to do battle with the frustrations that create anxiety. And the greater or more frequent the intake of food, the more it adds to body weight, hence obesity.

But something bizarre happens: the abnormally high intake of food with the intention, conscious or otherwise, of reducing anxiety and perhaps enhancing acceptance by the outside world has just the opposite effect. It increases the probability of rejections, due plainly to an ungainly appearance.

The traditional example of the fat girl is well known: she does not have a satisfactory social life, and spends her evenings home because few people ask for her company. She stays home—and eats candy—becomes fatter—decreases her chances for social relations—therewith eats more—further decreasing her opportunities.

The chain of evidence leading to the causes of obesity is primarily psychological. Most people overeat for psychological reasons. There is a way to correct obesity, but it is best to prevent it. The correction of obesity rests on two pillars, (1) caloric restriction and (2) psychological reevaluation. Both must be present to reduce weight and, above all, to keep it reduced. We shall discuss the details later.

While it is said that fat people do not want to reduce, consciously or not, they cannot or should not be blamed or condemned for their obesity, as fat does serve an inner psychological need. Successful weight reduction is obtained by the reevaluation of the psychological need served by fat or by the process of its acquisition. Restriction of caloric intake without a more basic insight into the reason for caloric over-acquisition will not have lasting benefits, because the obese person on a weight-reducing diet will not stick to it long.

Another difficulty found with weight reduction is based on the fact that food is also a cultural phenomenon. The dinner or feast as a cultural or religious event is well known. It is considered socially gauche to refuse to partake of food orgies, which many festive occasions represent. In the family matrix, the same cultural or social phenomenon takes place when a family celebrates an event.

In addition, there come into play the psychodynamics of family interaction. For example, a mother will frequently urge, implore, scream, in her attempts to push food into her children. Her basic reason is not nutritional concern. She may not be aware that she is not a loving mother. She stuffs her children with food to substitute for the love that she cannot give them—because she may not have it. A seductive or manipulative mother also uses food, among other devices, to gain her ends. The foundation for obesity is thus set for the children. They now have a solid background for the practice of excessive food intake in their adult years. Then, as a substitute for loneliness, for fatigue, for boredom, for an inner feeling of emptiness, they find temporary surcease by filling up with food. And many fears are born of loneliness, fatigue, boredom, emptiness; the attempt to assuage fear by food intake is well known.

Another important insight is that the same stimuli that

trigger people to gain weight may also cause a drastic and pathological loss of weight. Obesity is only one end of a spectrum. The other end is a condition called *anorexia nervosa,* which literally means lack of appetite due to nervous reasons. As with many other medical terms (hypersplenism, intermittent claudication, etc.), it does not give an explanation but is merely descriptive. In anorexia nervosa, which is usually found in adolescent girls, though it does also occur in other women, there is no desire to eat. Food intake is minimal, and body weight can drop drastically. Much as obesity, it is a disturbance of food intake. Thus obesity and anorexia nervosa are both horns of a dilemma—the Scylla and Charybdis of eating—and both have a psychological origin. In fact, it is not extraordinary, though not frequent, for people to go from one extreme to the other, if they survive it. Dietary and psychological ministrations treat both horns of the dilemma, obesity and anorexia nervosa—in obesity, dietary restriction; in anorexia nervosa, dietary plenty.

Extremely rapid reduction of body weight, which unfortunately is what the fat person wants, can precipitate a psychosis if not anorexia nervosa. Thus the *rate* of weight reduction is important in treating both obesity and anorexia nervosa.

One of the important concomitants to obesity is the feeling of being filled—satiety. An obese person has a hunger which he always attempts to sate. But two elements disturb this simple attempt: first, the hunger is not necessarily for food, though he attempts to sate it with food, and second, he is almost never sated. In fact the fat person may actually rarely be either hungry or full. He eats despite the fact that the hunger does not originate in the stomach but in the psyche. The thin person is easily sated, and perhaps therefore remains at a more-or-less constant weight.

While the body is growing, as during childhood and adolescence, there is a clear need to take in more food than is expended for energy. The rest is used for body growth—construction. After full growth is attained, the body is physiologically in a constant state; it does not need to grow. Thus, except for minor adjustments due to ongoing physiological processes, the body weight is and should remain constant. When the food intake is larger than necessary, the rest is stored. But the unfortunate point is that the excess is stored in the form of fat. The body has an almost unlimited capacity to store fat, contrary to its ability to store proteins and carbohydrates. The grand idea of caloric restriction is based on the fact that the stored fat can be used to produce energy needed for daily endeavors during the period that the food intake is smaller than the daily energy needed. It is fortunate that fat can be mobilized to take the place of food, and thus body fat can be lost. This is precisely what is necessary to reduce body weight.

But here is a caution: many people, especially women, would rather talk about reducing weight than actually reducing it. Weight reduction is a fashionable subject to talk about. Often, especially with people who are shy in starting a conversation with strangers, talk about fat reduction breaks the ice. *But it does not take off fat!* And with some, whose inner resources may be rather flat, or whose external interests are rather shallow, it remains one of the few subjects on which they can hold forth in confidence. This is also a factor in self-protection and an attempt to ward off anxiety: the talker-but-not-the-doer should not be blamed.

People usually welcome reasons other than overeating to account for their obesity. It is less than sociably acceptable to admit to overeating, but there is no social unacceptability to being fat due to "glands." As a matter of fact, there are only a few rather far-reaching metabolic causes of obesity, though they are rare. One of them is Cushing's syndrome, a disturbance of the adrenal-pituitary axis. Another is castration, male or female. A third is removal of the frontal lobes of the brain, prefrontal lobotomy. And weight gain frequently follows menopause. But even in the normal events of menopause, weight does not need to be gained if the caloric intake is reduced—often easier said than done.

Obesity has also been produced in rats by obliteration of a certain part of the brain (hypothalamus), after which they eat continuously. Most interestingly, obliteration of another part gives rise to such a lack of appetite that the rats actually starve in the midst of readily available food. This may or may not apply to humans. These centers in the brain are referred to as the appetite or hunger centers. But for all practical purposes, obesity in man is due to excessive food intake, not to destruction of part of the brain, though the reason for the superfluous food intake lies somewhere in the psyche.

How to reduce? To ask an obese person to use will power is naive. The matter is deeper. To ask him to stop eating is absurd. It does not touch the reason for overeating. To shame him into reducing is cruel; it is pointless and merely adds insult to injury. To give him a diet without psychological support is usually ineffective. To give him motivation is excellent, provided that his psychological constellation accepts it and that a substitute for the urge to overeat is also given. To tell him to go to a psychiatrist may justifiably produce a counterresponse to tell you to go to hell.

But there is hope. You can reduce and what is even more important, you can retain the new weight or the reduced status. Several instruments are necessary. One is a full-length mirror. Another is clothes—a dress or a suit *which has become too small.* But above all, the most important is your own conviction that loss of weight is imperative.

A scale is not necessary; in fact it may be a detriment. The reason that a scale is a liability is that if the loss of weight, as seen on a scale, is not quick or dramatic, people may become discouraged and relapse. They *see* no positive reinforcement, though it is there. Like drug addicts they relapse when the world does not embrace them for a small accomplishment. Yet even a small accomplishment is a sizable asset because it is a harbinger of the future.

The use of a full-length mirror in the nude, for which there is no substitute, accomplishes several ends. It allows you to take stock not only of your nude appearance but also of the distortions of your posture brought on by the excess weight. The distortion of form can become grotesque even with as little as 20 pounds overweight. But in assessing your appearance before a full-length mirror, do not draw in your abdomen or pose, as for a photograph. The worst delusion is self-delusion.

Also, a mirror, but only a full-length mirror, allows you to see progress in a more telling way than a scale does. A scale offers merely numbers, elements which have to be translated by the imagination. A full-length mirror can show you how both posture and form are improving—and how appearance is enhanced. That is positive reinforcement and will keep motivation on a workable level.

A suit or a dress that was at one time comfortable and now too small is a considerable help. While it cannot be worn every day, it should be put on every week, for comfortably fitting into clothes that were too small for you offers a much more satisfactory reward for reducing, as well as a stimulant to continue, than a scale.

For motivation there is no substitute. If you really want to reduce, rather than just talk about reducing, you have to be sold on the enduring advantage that results from eating less. For example, while it is known that fat people have a shorter life expectancy, you may not be impressed by that; it is too ephemeral to worry about events 20, 30, or 40 years hence.

But you may prize the advantages that an attractive weight will give you while you are in your prime of life. You may find it worthwhile to curtail food intake in exchange for gaining self-confidence (fat people are inevitably self-conscious), or for a better body-image of yourself, or for social acceptability, or even for the banal ability of climbing a flight of steps without the breathlessness that is associated with old age. Or you may want to break the patterns by which you have been enslaved in other areas. If you are fat, that is a splendid way to start.

In any event, the motivation must come from within. We shall not go into the various aspects of physiological health or mental health that weight reduction brings. You may have known them, even vaguely. But if you were not moved by these reasons in the past, no matter how compelling they are, it was due to the fact that you may have had little motivation to reduce body weight.

Should you develop motivation within, you should also be

aware of the obstacles that may be in your way; awareness is the first part of victory. For example, if you work at home, or you are a housewife, the temptation to eat is greater, no matter how busy you are. You may find that a change, such as part-time work outside of the house, makes the first few weeks or months easier to implement or to effect your motivation. At times other events in the familial structure conspire against you and you put on weight. For example, children going to college out-of-town or the death of a spouse may be instrumental in gaining weight. Adjustment, by occupation outside of the house, may be the answer to assuaging the frustration or the hollowness produced by such changes.

What may be on the surface an imperceptible change can lead to weight increase. Awareness is necessary here. For example, a reduction of activity such as the installation of a

Desirable Weights

Weight in Pounds According to Frame (In Indoor Clothing)

MEN OF AGES 25 AND OVER

Height (with shoes on) 1-inch heels Feet	Inches	*Small Frame*	*Medium Frame*	*Large Frame*
5	2	112–120	118–129	126–141
5	3	115–123	121–133	129–144
5	4	118–126	124–136	132–148
5	5	121–129	127–139	135–152
5	6	124–133	130–143	138–156
5	7	128–137	134–147	142–161
5	8	132–141	138–152	147–166
5	9	136–145	142–156	151–170
5	10	140–150	146–160	155–174
5	11	144–154	150–165	159–179
6	0	148–158	154–170	164–184
6	1	152–162	158–175	168–189
6	2	156–167	162–180	173–194
6	3	160–171	167–185	178–199
6	4	164–175	172–190	182–204

labor-saving device may lead to an increase in weight. Another example: it was found that typists in the pool of a large corporation gained weight in a four-month period after their manual typewriters were changed to electric ones.

Awareness must also be used in the attempt to add exercise to the sedentary person's weight-reducing regimen. For example, there is a *net gain* in weight if two cocktails are taken after an 18-hole game of golf, which uses about 140 calories of energy expenditure. Two cocktails are equivalent to about 175 calories—a net caloric gain.

Do not ignore the small amount of daily calories that are waiting for you in snacks ready to pounce on you. Always multiply the caloric value by 365, the number of days in the year. For example, only 100 calories a day of some goody amount to 36,500 calories a year—about 9 pounds of fat!

WOMEN OF AGES 25 AND OVER

Height (with shoes on) 2-inch heels Feet	Inches	*Small Frame*	*Medium Frame*	*Large Frame*
4	10	92– 98	96–107	104–119
4	11	94–101	98–110	106–122
5	0	96–104	101–113	109–125
5	1	99–107	104–116	112–128
5	2	102–110	107–119	115–131
5	3	105–113	110–122	118–134
5	4	108–116	113–126	121–138
5	5	111–119	116–130	125–142
5	6	114–123	120–135	129–146
5	7	118–127	124–139	133–150
5	8	122–131	128–143	137–154
5	9	126–135	132–147	141–158
5	10	130–140	136–151	145–163
5	11	134–144	140–155	149–168
6	0	138–148	144–159	153–173

For girls between 18 and 25, subtract 1 pound for each year under 25.

Courtesy of Metropolitan Life Insurance Co.

In this connection note the reverse too. While walking is not a dramatic way of reducing—you need to walk 35 miles to reduce one pound of *fat*—it totals up in the course of a year. Daily exercise does reduce weight over the long term, aside from its other benefits.

We shall not set forth a dietary scheme. Lists and books on caloric values and other food values are readily obtainable.

But we want to point out some common practices and to evaluate them. If food is a sedative, and that sedative value will be lost due to caloric restriction, people often take alcohol to "settle down," to unwind. The fallacy here lies in the fact that alcohol contains 7 calories per gram, while proteins and carbohydrates contain only 4 calories per gram. Alcohol is exceeded in caloric value only by fat, which is equivalent to 9 calories per gram. Moreover, alcohol is both a nervous system depressant and an appetite stimulant. Alcohol gives you empty calories. As a substitute, chew on a carrot or on celery, dipped in a dry wine, *not* a sweet wine with its higher (20%) alcoholic content. Dry wines contain less sugar and have an alcoholic content of 10% to 12%. Remember, too, that alcohol has no satiety value.

In choosing a diet remember that you want to reduce predominantly fat, not muscle. Hence, be sure to have a diet that is high in protein. One gram of protein per day is required per 2.2 pounds (1 kg.) of desired body weight. The high-protein diets with very low carbohydrates are effective, at least for a limited time, until a dietary adjustment has taken place.

People eat more during cold weather or after exposure to cold. The reason is that the heat loss, hence energy loss, is greater and an attempt to make it up may lead to excessive food consumption. If you are cold, and you need to warm up from inside out, a clear, nonfat broth, or hot coffee or tea (not hot chocolate) will serve the purpose much more efficiently than food.

In devising your reducing diet you must take into consideration certain factors such as the satiety value of foods (to reduce the feeling of emptiness) in addition to their nutritional value. Fats and proteins sate more easily, hence have a high satiety value; carbohydrates have a smaller satiety value, and alcohol has none! Therefore, some fats with proteins are advisable.

Foods that have a high bulk or residue value are found by some to satisfy the empty feeling. For example, assuming that the caloric values of white bread and whole wheat bread are the same (there is only a small difference), white bread has much less residue than whole wheat bread. So make whatever little bread you eat whole wheat bread.

There is virtually no restriction on the kind of meat as a protein source. But in the attempt to enhance protein intake do not go overboard on eggs, as they are high in cholesterol. You will find that canned raw sauerkraut is an ideal low-calorie roughage producer—a grand pacifier for the empty feeling. It contains only 22 calories per 100 grams (about 3⅓ oz.). If you prefer it boiled, that is fine; but do not make the error of preparing an old-fashioned cooked sauerkraut dish which contains potatoes, peas or lentils, bacon and meat scraps.

Cabbage has about the same caloric and roughage value as sauerkraut. But it has a mild irritating quality and may increase appetite. As snacks or as a dish you will find the following to be low in calories and quite filling: cooked turnips 27, raw spinach 20, raw mushrooms 16, canned mushrooms 11. (The foregoing figures refer to the number of calories per 100 grams, equivalent to about 3⅓ oz., which is a generous portion.) But be aware, as the following "innocent" vegetables pack a caloric wallop: dry peas 344, dry lentils 340, lima beans 335—all calories per 100 grams.

Salads are a treat and also a hidden danger. They add needed roughage to the calorie-restricted diet but can undo the good work by a glob of salad dressing. We agree that vinegar alone makes the salad unappetizing. Lemon is better. A teaspoonful of yogurt may be a good substitute for salad dressing—if you like it. You will find, however, that a liberal sprinkling of such spices as tarragon, dill, basil, rosemary, sage, nutmeg, curry, sesame, anise, fennel or caraway seeds, mustard, chili make a salad appetizing. Or you may even douse a salad with vinegar in which one or two of these spices were soaked for some days. You may find these spices to be a new taste sensation which can be used without guilt. (The only exception is chili or mustard, which should be used sparingly as they are irritating and can increase appetite.)

Ordinarily, salt does not have to be omitted, but it is a good idea to reduce it. Salt binds water in the tissues. Catsup, pickles, Worcestershire and similar sauces are also high in salt.

Another form of caloric restriction is the *omnidiet* (*omni* = all). By this device, while eating your normal diet, you observe only two restrictions: (1) you eat your normal diet but you consume only half the quantity you normally eat, and (2) you eliminate *all* alcohol and you further cut down to a very minimum any potatoes and bread from the half-portions you are now eating. This is an effective form of dietary control, and perhaps a less trying one, because the change is not as drastic, and includes most of the familiar foods you normally consume.

The slow reduction of weight is a more satisfying one because there is less discomfort and a greater likelihood of continuing it. Hence, relapses are perhaps less likely. More particularly, slow reduction of body weight will allow your skin to adjust to the new shape; there will be less hanging of folds of skin.

A form of do-it-yourself dietary control that is eminently effective is the aversion method. This is probably based upon Oscar Wilde's quip that "To think a thing is to cause it to be," or perhaps more likely William James's epigrammatic "Believe, and your belief will help create the fact."

The aversion method merely requires the user to look upon food with disgust. It is really not hard to do. Using this approach, a person will eat part of the dish set before him, but will leave the rest. This may well be a more sound method, because obesity is basically caused by a psychically triggered urge to acquire food. Hence, a psychically conditioned sense of disgust should counterbalance the acquisitive urge.

Since in any regimen for reducing body weight dietary

intake is reduced, a high-potency multivitamin tablet should be taken daily to prevent a vitamin deficiency.

You have heard of starvation diets. They are enticing regimens for almost instant weight reduction. Under certain conditions they may be desirable, but they must be undertaken only in a hospital under the direct supervision of a physician. And they have substantial drawbacks or dangers.

One drawback is that such rapid loss of weight does not allow the elasticity of the skin to adjust to the new contour. The result: skin hangs on the body in an unsightly way. Another drawback is that muscle as well as fat is lost, which can be a metabolically serious development. Other undesirable effects are acidosis or ketosis and loss of valuable electrolytes.

Another drawback, a more serious one, is the possibility that a psychosis may be precipitated. In fact, psychosis is an ever present danger in a starvation diet. This is not surprising, in view of the fact that obesity is broadly considered the result of neurotic behavior. That is the reason that psychological support and unmistakable self-motivation are as important as dietary restriction for enduring effects.

Perhaps the most effective form of obesity treatment is group therapy, provided that the individual (1) is highly motivated, (2) has found an acceptable group, and (3) is in the care of an acceptable therapist.

Obesity is a national problem of malnutrition. It exceeds any other aspect of malnutrition in the number of individuals affected. Obesity as well as starvation are dysfunctions of nutrition.

There are few contraindications to reducing obesity due to fat. One is tuberculosis, because it is believed—though by no means certain—that reduction of body weight may reactivate a latent and quiescent case of tuberculosis infection. Perhaps this point is moot because few seriously ill tuberculous individuals are overweight. People who are obese, and have a serious disease—as tuberculosis, heart disease, etc.—should not reduce without the clear advice of their physician.

There are no other conditions in which excessive weight should not be reduced.

INGREDIENTS

No drug products, either those available on prescription or over-the-counter without prescription, reduce weight. At best they reduce the desire to eat, and only restriction of dietary intake reduces body weight. None of the products sold as an aid to weight reduction are useful without dietary restriction and without motivation. They may, however, make it easier for a highly motivated person.

Reducing products, as they are commonly called, must be taken with caution, not because they are dangerous—though some can be—but because reliance on them may prevent an individual from seeking more competent methods of weight reduction.

Some of the products available over-the-counter without prescription, as Metrecal, are actually foods. Their advantage in a weight-reduction regimen lies in the fact that by taking them you can precisely measure your caloric intake provided that you conform to directions given. Such products supply proteins, carbohydrates and fats, to assure adequate nutrition, with vitamins and minerals to supplement those which are missing from a restricted diet. In many cases, the total daily food intake consists of these preparations. Variants of these preparations are in cookie form.

The disadvantage of these products lies in the fact that though they are palatable, the sensory component of food intake is missing. Thus early relapse to the regular and unsatisfactory diet is more likely. Some people, however, completely misunderstand the premise on which these preparations are used, and take twice or three times the amounts recommended. The net result is they *gain* weight instead of losing it.

Another type of weight-reducing product consists of wafers with a diet pamphlet. These wafers are high in protein and low in fat, and together with the dietary information and dietary restriction they may be helpful to a strongly motivated person—if it works for him.

An additional form of over-the-counter weight-reducing

product consists of candy which contains vitamins and some minerals, notably iron. The principle inherent in this type of product is that candy satisfies, helps sate the user on a reducing diet (about three pieces a day are recommended), and prevents the urge to take more caloric foods. Each piece of candy is high in carbohydrates, moderate in fat and low in protein, and contains 26 calories. If it is found that one, and only one, piece of candy prevents taking more caloric foods—then well and good. But motivation is what gives the successful dieter power to conform to a reducing diet.

Then there is the product in the form of chewing gum or a tablet, which, containing a local anesthetic, benzocaine, is said to reduce the sensory desire for food or to cut down the quantity of its intake. The objective is to substitute one sensation with another, the latter one not leading to caloric intake. These tablets are highly flavored and as with slimming candy, if this method prevents you from yearning for more food or dessert, well and good. But motivation still is the real answer.

A further method offered by a group of over-the-counter preparations available without prescription is a combination in tablet form of phenylpropanolamine hydrochloride, with vitamins, at times with caffeine, and occasionally with methylcellulose. None of these, of course, will work without dietary restriction. The vitamins are to substitute those which are lost because of dietary restriction. The caffeine is a stimulant, which is needed because curtailment of food intake tends to depress. But there is too little caffeine (25 mg.) present for that purpose. Methyl cellulose swells in the intestine to give a feeling of bulk to assuage the empty feeling. The trouble is that the place you need it more is in the stomach.

The more important ingredient in these preparations is phenylpropanolamine hydrochloride. Similar to ephedrine, phenylpropanolamine finds its most widespread and dependable uses as an ingredient in nasal or sinus congestion. But one of its actions, though a mild one, is depression of appetite, for which reason it is used in these preparations. The effect is probably too mild in the 25 mg. doses administered. But in larger doses it could produce palpitations or wakefulness, and then it would not be available over-the-counter without prescription. Its inclusion in these products is logical, but the degree of the functional effect in reducing appetite may vary from individual to individual. Surely, without caloric restriction it would be useless. No drug is known that takes off fat without causing substantial metabolic upheavals.

An additional method of weight reduction does lessen body weight but not fat; it is a diuretic causing water loss by increasing the flow of urine. *A diuretic does not reduce fat.* Do not consider these products. If you have an accumulation of water in the tissues (edema) see your doctor; it may be due to a dysfunctioning heart.

Though not available without prescription, we should mention thyroid, which is reputed to be weight reducing. If the thyroid is normal, thyroid tablets will reduce weight only in doses that will be toxic, and which can damage the heart. As a matter of fact, one is worse off after having taken thyroid tablets, whether they reduce or not, because thyroid tablets suppress the natural function of the thyroid gland in the body. The thyroid gland recovers its function—with time. In the event of an underfunction of the thyroid (hypothyroidism) other problems, perhaps more than weight gain, will be present. They should be treated by a physician.

A group of products that create bulk in the intestine—for which reason they are used in constipation—are the hydrophylic colloids, or bulk-producing agents. Creating bulk in the intestine may be helpful when it gives an intestinal sense of fullness. But the sense of fullness is more necessary in the stomach where hunger contractions take place. For some people, however, but with dietary measures, they may be helpful. (They are listed under Laxatives; see pages 85–86 for names of products.)

As a sweetener saccharin is almost universally used. Cyclamates are no longer available, by government fiat. But some people complain that saccharin leaves a bad aftertaste, yet they do not like unsweetened beverages. The aftertaste can be easily remedied by using only half of that amount of saccharin which was found to be unpleasant. In a short time, perhaps in a week or two, you will become accustomed to and satisfied with partially sweetened beverages.

If Your Need Is for a Product Against Obesity:

Look for Products Containing the Following Ingredients:
Bulk-forming agents which can be useful to allay hunger pangs.
Avoid the Following Ingredients:
Diuretics (they do not reduce fat)
Amphetamines

NAMES OF PRODUCTS

Ayds Reducing Plan—Vitamin/Mineral Candy (Campana Corp.)—Candy or fudge of different types, containing the common vitamins and minerals, including iron. Each piece of candy is equivalent to 26 calories and contains 3.2% protein, 74.7% carbohydrate, and 9.2% fat.

Dietene (Doyle)—A powder containing 33% protein, 0.7% fat, and 53% carbohydrates, vitamins and minerals, from which milk shakes are made, to be used in conjunction with a stated 1,000 calorie reducing diet, which provides (*including* two Dietene shakes), 81 gm. protein, 30 gm. fat, and 105 gm. carbohydrates.

Di-Ette Reducing Plan (Standard-American Products Corp.)—Contains phenylpropanolamine hydrochloride, caffeine, methyl cellulose (quantities not listed on label), and vitamins.

Diurex Pills (Amco)—Contains buchu, methylene blue, oil juniper, theobromine, potassium salicylate and uva ursi. Offered as a diuretic. Does not reduce fat.

Fluitabs (Hall)—Contains extracts of buchu, uva-ursi, corn silk, juniper, and caffeine. Offered as a diuretic to dispose of accumulation of water in the tissues—weak at that. Does *not* reduce fat.

Melozets Methyl Cellulose Wafers (Quinton/Merck)—Each wafer contains 1.5 gm. methyl cellulose, with wheat flour base, equivalent to 30 calories each. Must be taken with water. Offered in conjunction with reducing diets to give bulk and reduce discomfort of hunger pangs.

Metrecal Cookies (Mead Johnson)—Cookies made of milk protein concentrate, sugar, wheat flour, hydrogenated vegetable shortening, vitamins and minerals, equivalent to 30% protein, 48%

carbohydrates, and 8% fat. Nine (9) cookies, the amount recommended for each meal, are equivalent to 225 calories, 17.5 gm. protein, 27.5 gm. carbohydrates, and 5 gm. fat.

Metrecal Powder (Mead Johnson) —A powder containing in each ½ lb. (4 scoopfuls) 70 gm. protein, 20 gm. fat, and 110 gm. carbohydrates (approximately 30% protein, 9% fat, 48% carbohydrates) equivalent to 900 calories, with vitamins and minerals. Made from nonfat dry milk, sugar, partially hydrogenated soy oil, and milk protein concentrate. A drink made according to directions (one scoopful and water to make 8 oz. liquid) is equivalent to 225 calories and is used in place of regular food or in place of a meal.

Metrecal Shape Liquid Diet Food (Mead Johnson) —A liquid containing in each 8 fluid oz. 16.25 gm. protein, 3 gm. fat, and 33.25 gm. carbohydrates (6.3% protein, 1.2% fat, 13% carbohydrates), equivalent to 225 calories, with vitamins and minerals. Made from concentrated skim milk, sugar, sodium caseinate, and partially hydrogenated soy oil. Used in place of regular food or in place of a meal.

Proslim (J. B. Williams) —Supplies a diet book showing a balanced menu for 7 days at 1,000 calories a day, with wafers, each 9.3 calories. Eight (8) wafers are recommended by the manufacturer per day, which contain 61% protein, 26% carbohydrates, and 2% fat. It is offered as a protein food and dietary system. Also available as a high-protein diet mix making a chocolate-flavored drink containing 40 calories per packet.

Slim-Mint (Thompson Medical Co.) —Tablets containing benzocaine, methyl cellulose, dextrose, and flavoring oils. Offered for use before meals, to obtund appetite, or after meals instead of dessert and with beverage.

X-11 Diet Plan Tablets (Porter & Dietsch) —Contains phenylpropanolamine hydrochloride, caffeine (quantities not listed on label), and vitamins.

UNDERWEIGHT

DEFINITION

Underweight is the opposite of obesity. The underweight person is one who weighs at least 10% less than the "normal" in height-frame-weight tables. (See chapter on obesity for tables.)

CAUSE

The reason for underweight may lie in diseases which can be serious, such as hyperthyroidism or tuberculosis, which need medical attention. However, we are concerned with underweight not related to disease conditions. Call it "simple" underweight. The reason for such underweight is due predominantly to the fact that food intake is smaller than the energy expenditure warrants.

DISCUSSION AND CAUTIONS

People are thin—thinner than what the tables list as average weight—because their caloric intake is too small to balance their energy expenditure. But they may be thinner because their individual metabolism does not fully utilize food. This may be due to certain dysfunctions of the gastrointestinal tract. These dysfunctions are conditions we are not discussing because they should be carefully treated by a physician. But some people are just simply thin, without other problems or conditions that require medical attention. We address ourselves to such a situation.

Why is it that these people, predominantly women, become conscious of their underweight when spring comes? Can it be due to their visualizing themselves in a bathing suit? Are they possibly concerned that their breasts are too small? And do they believe that if they gain weight their breasts will increase in size?

Here is something to bear in mind: the angular shape, narrow hips, small breasts, of an underweight female, or a nonrounded shape (low feminine profile), will not improve with weight gain. Nor will small breasts become distinctly larger. That is a matter of endocrinological development, and such conditions are best given attention by an endocrinologist.

But if these problems are not present, and you want to gain weight—say, 10 to 15 pounds—you may do so by increasing your caloric intake. This is most efficiently done by a diet high in fat, because fat intake is the most economic and efficient way of gaining weight. But do not overload with fat by eating a bar of butter like a bar of candy! The load on digestion would be unduly heavy. Instead, a nutritionally balanced diet, relatively high in fat, is desirable. Such a diet should include the usual proteins and carbohydrates but also a quart of milk daily, which is equivalent to somewhat more than 660 calories. Cheese and organ meats are also rich in fat. Many desserts, while not necessarily rich in fat, are high in carbohydrates and should be curtailed. A table of such food values is readily obtainable.

As people age they normally lose weight. This may be due to a combination of lessened food absorption, but predominantly tissue fat and water are lost as aging continues.

PRODUCTS

Since a market exists for products that add body weight, they have been made available. Some, like Sustagen, are predominantly for adding calories and nutritive value during convalescence and under other conditions in which a high caloric intake is desirable. Others are made available to supply the demand for *fat tablets*. As to the economics involved: you will find that calorie for calorie, food may be less expensive and give greater sensory pleasure.

If Your Need Is for a Product Against Underweight:

Look for Products Containing the Following Ingredients:

- Fats
- Carbohydrates
- Proteins

NAMES OF PRODUCTS

Meritene (Doyle)—Contains skim milk solids, maltodextrins, lecithin, essential vitamins, iron, and traces of iodine. Equivalent to 33% protein, 0.2% fat, and 58% carbohydrates.

Sustagen (Mead Johnson)—Contains skim milk solids, dextrins, dextrose, maltose (Dextri-Maltose), powdered whole milk, calcium caseinate, essential vitamins, and iron. Equal parts of Sustagen and water make 50 calories per fluid ounce. Each pound contains 105 gm. protein (approximately 23%) and 1,750 calories.

Wate On Tablets (Fleetwood)—Tablets containing whole milk powder, tricalcium phosphate, dextrose, monoglycerides and diglycerides, vitamins, and minerals. Twelve (12) tablets with one quart of milk (4 glasses of 8 oz. each) supply 920 calories. Since a quart of milk supplies 664 calories, 12 tablets are equivalent to 256 calories, an expensive form of caloric intake.

Wate On Tablets, New Fortified Formula (Fleetwood)—Tablets containing vegetable fat, sodium caseinate, sugar, dicalcium phosphate, salt, vitamins, and minerals. Three (3) tablets with a glass of milk supply 205 calories. Since a glass (8 oz.) of milk alone supplies 166 calories, the 3 tablets supply 39 calories. This new fortified formula supplies a smaller caloric intake than the regular Wate On tablets, and is an even more expensive form of caloric intake.

APPENDIX A

LIST OF SYNONYMS OR OTHER NAMES

In most cases in the general discussions we refer to the chemical, official, or established name of the ingredients in the products discussed, and only give those rather than their trade name. Our reason for doing so is to avoid an implication of favoring a given product. Nonetheless, some trade names are more commonly known and are more easily remembered.

For easy reference, the following is a list of names by which certain ingredients or products are also known and by which they can be recognized. This information has been given in the previous individual lists of products, but the reader may find it convenient to see it all grouped in one place, if all he wants to do is to look up a certain ingredient and ascertain a trade name that contains it.

To simplify further, only the basic name of the ingredient is given, such as *phenylephrine* rather than *phenylephrine hydrochloride*. Though many of the substances given in the list below are available in the form of salts, such as hydrochlorides, hydrobromides, sulfates, maleates, etc., it makes little difference to the reader which salt is used, and may only complicate the name were we to add the specific salt name, as hydrochloride, etc. (Capitalized names are trade names.)

acetaminophen: APAP; Tempra; Tylenol; Valadol.
acetphenolisatin: oxyphenisatin; diacetyldiphenolisatin; Isacen.
ammoniated mercury: ammoniated mercuric chloride.
benzalkonium chloride: Zephiran Chloride; Zephirol; Roccal; Germitol; alkyldimethyl benzylammonium chloride.

benzethonium chloride: Phemerol; Quatrachlor; Solamine; Hyamine 1622.
benzocaine: ethyl aminobenzoate.
bisacodyl: Dulcolax; Durolax.
butacaine: Butesin.
carbamide: urea.
carbetapentane: Toclase.
casanthranol: Cantralax.
cetyldimethylbenzylammonium chloride: cetalkonium chloride.
cetylpyridinium: Ceepryn; Cepacol.
cetyltrimethylammonium bromide: cetrimonium bromide; Cetavlon; C.T.A.B.
chloroxylenol: 4-chloro-3,5-xylenol; parachlorometaxylenol; *p*-chlor-*m*-xylenol.
chlorpheniramine: Chlor-Trimeton.
cyclomethycaine: Surfacaine; Topocaine.
danthron: 1-8-dihydroxyanthraquinone; Dorbane.
dequalinium: decamine.
diamthazole: Asterol.
dibucaine: Nupercaine.
dicyclomine: Bentyl.
dihydroxyacetone: Protosol.
dimenhydrinate: Dramamine.
dioctyl sodium sulfosuccinate: DOSS; DSS; Aerosol OT; Colace; Doxinate.
dioxybenzone: 2,2′-dihydroxy-4-methoxybenzophenone; Spectra-Sorb UV 24.
diperodon: Diothane.
diphenhydramine: Benadryl.
doxylamine: Decapryn.
2-ethoxyethyl-*p*-methoxycinnamate: Giv-Tan.
hexachlorophene: G-11; AT-7; Gamophen; Hexosan; pHisohex.
hexylresorcinol: Sucrets; S.T.37.
8-hydroxyquinoline: Quinophenol; Bioquin; oxyquinoline.
isooctylphenoxypolyethanol: Triton.
lidocaine: Xylocaine; lignocaine.
menthol: 3-*p*-menthanol; 1-menthol; hexahydrothymol; peppermint camphor.
mercury: quicksilver.
methapyrilene: Thenylene; Semikon; Histadyl; Dormin.
methoxyphenamine: Orthoxine.

methylbenzethonium chloride: Diaparene; Hyamine 10X.
methylparaben: Tegosept M; methyl parasept.
monobenzone: monobenzyl ether of hydroquinone; Benoquin; Benzoquin.
naphazoline: Privine.
nonylphenol surfactant: Igepal, a variety of.
octylphenoxypolyethoxyethanol: Igepal, a variety of; Antarox, a variety of.
orthophenylphenol: Dowicide 1.
oxybenzone: 2-hydroxy-4-methoxybenzophenone; Spectra-Sorb UV 9.
oxyphenisatin: acetphenolisatin; endophenolphthalein; Isacen; diacetyldiphenolisatin.
oxyquinoline: 8-hydroxyquinoline; Quinophenol; Bioquin.
papain: Caroid.
***para*-aminobenzoic acid:** 4-aminobenzoic acid; PABA; *p*-aminobenzoic acid.
parachlorometaxylenol: chloroxylenol; 4-chloro-3,5-xylenol; *p*-chlor-*m*-xylenol.
phenacetin: acetphenetidin.
phenindamine: Thephorin.
pheniramine: Trimeton; Inhiston.
phenol: carbolic acid; phenyl hydroxide; hydroxybenzene; oxybenzene.
beta-phenoxyethyldodecyldimethylammonium bromide: Domiphen; PDDB; Bradosol.
phenylephrine: Neo-Synephrine; Isophrin.
phenylmercuric nitrate: merphenyl nitrate.
phenylpropanolamine: Propadrine; *dl*-norephedrine.
phenyltoloxamine: Phenoxadrine; Bristamin.
plantago seeds: psyllium.
polyethylene lauryl alcohol: Brij, a variety of.
polyoxyethylene lauryl ether: Brij, a variety of.
polyoxyethylene nonylphenol: Triton, a variety of.
polyoxyethylene sorbitan monooleate: Tween 80; polysorbate 80; Monitan.
povidone-iodine: Isodine; PVP; Betadine; Proviodine.
pramoxine: Tronothane.
propylhexedrine: Benzedrex.
pyrilamine: Neo-Antergan.
selenium sulfide: Selsun.
simethicone: dimethicone; Antifoam A Compound; Mylicon.

sodium lauryl sulfate: Irium; dodecyl sodium sulfate; Duponol C; Gardinol.

sodium octylphenoxyethoxyethylether sulfonate: Entsufon.

stearyl dimethyl benzylammonium chloride: Triton, a variety of.

sulisobenzone: 2-hydroxy-4-methoxybenzophenone-5-sulfonic acid; Spectra-Sorb UV 284.

tetracaine: Pontocaine; Amethocaine.

tetrahydrozoline: Tyzine; Visine.

thenyldiamine: Thenfadil.

thonzylamine: Anahist; Neohetramine; Novohetramin.

tolnaftate: Tinactin; Tonoftal.

tripelennamine: Pyribenzamine; PBZ.

tyloxapol: Superinone.

xylometazoline: Otrivin.

APPENDIX B

SIDE EFFECTS OF CERTAIN INGREDIENTS

The Federal Food, Drug, and Cosmetic Act requires that certain ingredients used in preparations available over-the-counter carry stipulated warnings. These warnings are generally intended to alert the consumer, to enable him to use over-the-counter products safely, or, in the event that certain side effects occur, to discontinue the use of these preparations.

The following is a list of those warnings:

Acetaminophen Do not give to children under 3 years of age or use for more than 10 days unless directed by a physician. If pain persists for more than 10 days, or redness is present, or in conditions affecting children under 12 years of age, consult a physician immediately.

Acetanilid Do not exceed recommended dosage. Overdosage or continued use may result in serious blood disturbances.

Acetphenetidin-Containing Preparations This medication may damage the kidneys when used in large amounts or for a long period of time. Do not take more than the recommended dosage, nor take regularly for longer than 10 days without consulting your physician.

Anesthetics for External Use (Local Anesthetics) Do not use in the eyes. Not for prolonged use. If the condition for which this preparation is used persists or if a rash or irritation develops, discontinue use and consult a physician.

Antihistaminics for External Use Do not use in the eyes. If the condition for which this preparation is used persists or if a rash or irritation develops, discontinue use and consult a physician.

Antihistaminics, Oral This preparation may cause drowsiness. Do not drive or operate machinery while taking this medication. Do not give to children under 6 years of age or exceed the recommended dosage unless directed by a physician. (The reference to drowsiness is not required on preparations for the promotion of sleep or on preparations that are shown not to produce drowsiness.)

Antiperspirants Do not apply to broken skin. If a rash develops, discontinue use.

Antiseptics for External Use In case of deep or puncture wounds or serious burns, consult a physician. If redness, irritation, swelling, or pain persists or increases or if infection occurs discontinue use and consult a physician. (The reference to wounds and burns is not required on preparations intended solely for diaper rash.)

Belladonna Preparations and Preparations of Its Alkaloids (Atropine, Hyoscyamine, and Scopolamine (Hyoscine): Hyoscyamus, Stramonium, and Related Drug Preparations Not to be used by elderly persons or by children under 6 years of age unless directed by a physician. Do not exceed recommended dosage. Not for frequent or prolonged use. If dryness of the mouth occurs, decrease dosage. Discontinue use if rapid pulse, dizziness, or blurring of vision occurs.

Boric Acid Do not use as a dusting powder, especially on infants, or take internally. Use only as a solution. Do not apply to badly broken or raw skin or to large areas of the body.

Bromides Use only as directed. Do not give to children or use in the presence of kidney disease. If skin rash appears or if nervous symptoms persist, recur frequently, or are unusual, discontinue use and consult a physician.

Carbolic Acid (Phenol) Preparations (More Than 0.5%) for External Use Use according to directions. Do not apply to large areas of the body. If applied to fingers or toes, do not bandage.

Cathartics and Laxatives—Irritants and Other Peristaltic Stimulants Do not use when abdominal pain, nausea, or vomiting is present. Frequent or prolonged use may result in dependence on laxatives. If skin rash appears, do not use any preparation containing phenolphthalein.

"Cough-Due-to-Cold" Preparations (Dextromethorphan Hydrobromide and Carbetapentane Citrate) Keep out of the reach of children. Do not administer to children under 2 years of age unless directed by a physician. Persistent cough may indicate the presence of a serious condition. Persons with a high fever or persistent cough should not use this preparation unless directed by a physician.

Counterirritants and Rubefacients (Liniments) Do not apply to irritated skin or if excessive irritation develops. Avoid getting into the eyes or on mucous membranes. If pain persists for more than 10 days, or redness is present, or in conditions affecting children under 12 years of age, consult a physician immediately.

Diamthazole Dihydrochloride for External Use Do not apply to children under 6 years of age because serious reactions may occur. Do not apply to children 6 to 12 years of age unless directed by a physician. Do not use on mucous membranes. Discontinue use and consult a physician if irritation develops or relief is not obtained. Keep out of the reach of children.

Diarrhea Preparations Do not use for more than 2 days or in the presence of high fever or in infants or children under 3 years of age unless directed by a physician.

Dicyclomine Hydrochloride with an Antacid Do not exceed the recommended dosage. Do not administer to children under 12 years of age or use for a prolonged period unless directed by a physician, since persistent or recurring symptoms may indicate a serious disease requiring medical attention.

Douche Preparations Do not use more often than twice weekly unless directed by a physician.

Dressings, Protective Spray-on Type In case of deep or puncture wounds or serious burns, consult a physician. If redness, irritation, swelling, or pain persists or increases or if infection occurs consult a physician. Keep away from eyes or other mucous membranes. Avoid inhaling.

Ephedrine Preparations (Oral) Do not exceed the recommended dosage. Reduce dosage if nervousness, restlessness, or sleeplessness occurs. Do not use if high blood pressure, heart disease, diabetes, or thyroid disease is present unless directed by a physician.

Epinephrine Inhalation 1:100 (Not for Injection) For inhalation only. Reduce dosage if bronchial irritation, nervousness, restlessness, or sleeplessness occurs. Do not use if high blood pressure, heart disease, diabetes, or thyroid disease is present unless directed by a physician. If prompt relief is not obtained consult a physician. Do not use epinephrine inhalation if it is brown in color or contains a precipitate.

Iodine and Iodides (Oral) If a skin rash appears, discontinue use and consult a physician.

Ipecac Syrup for Emergency Treatment of Poisoning, to Induce Vomiting Before using, call a physician, the Poison Control Center, or a hospital emergency room immediately for advice. Keep out of reach of children. Do not use in unconscious persons. Ordinarily, this drug should not be used if strychnine, corrosives such as alkalies (lye) and strong acids, or petroleum distillates such as kerosine, gasoline, coal oil, fuel oil, paint thinner, or cleaning fluid have been ingested.

Mercury Preparations for External Use Discontinue use if rash or irritation develops or if the condition for which used persists. Frequent or prolonged use or application to large areas may cause serious mercury poisoning.

Ammoniated mercury bleach cream: Discontinue use if rash or irritation develops. Do not apply to irritated or damaged skin (cuts, bruises, sunburn) or after shaving or using a depilatory. Do not apply to children under 12 years of age.

Mineral Oil Laxatives Take only at bedtime. Avoid prolonged use. Do not administer to infants or young children, in pregnancy, or to bedridden or aged patients unless directed by a physician.

Nasal Preparations: Oil Base Do not exceed recommended dosage nor use for prolonged period. Do not administer to infants or children unless directed by a physician. Do not use as a spray.

Nasal Preparations in Plastic Spray Containers Avoid overdosage. Follow directions for use carefully.

Nasal Preparations: Vasoconstrictors (Ephedrine, epinephrine, Methamphetamine, and Others of Similar Activity) Do not exceed recommended dosage. Overdosage may cause nervousness, restlessness, or sleeplessness. Do not use for more than 3 or 4 consecutive days unless directed by a physician.

Ophthalmic Preparations If irritation persists or increases, discontinue use and consult a physician. Keep container tightly closed. Do not touch dropper tip to any surface, since this may contaminate solution.

Phenylephrine Hydrochloride Preparations, Oral Individuals with high blood pressure, heart disease, diabetes, or thyroid disease should use only as directed by a physician.

Phenylpropanolamine Hydrochloride Preparations, Oral Individuals with high blood pressure, heart disease, diabetes, or thyroid disease should use only as directed by a physician.

Rectal Preparations for External Use In case of rectal bleeding, consult your physician promptly.

Resorcinol (Not the Monoacetate) Hair Preparations Excessive use of this preparation may temporarily discolor blond, white, or red hair.

Salicylates, Including Aspirin and Salicylamide (Except Methyl Salicylate, Effervescent Salicylate Preparations, and Preparations of Aminosalicylic Acid and Its Salts) Keep these and *all* medicines out of children's reach. In case of accidental overdose, contact a physician immediately.

For children under 3 years of age, consult your physician. If pain persists for more than 10 days, or redness is present, or in conditions affecting children under 12 years of age, consult a physician immediately.

Salicylates: Methyl Salicylate (Wintergreen Oil) Do not use other than as directed. Keep out of the reach of children to avoid accidental poisoning. If the preparation is a counterirritant or rubefacient, discontinue use if excessive irritation of the skin develops. Avoid getting into the eyes or on mucous membranes. If pain persists for more than 10 days, or redness is present, or in conditions affecting children under 12 years of age, consult a physician immediately.

Scopolamine Preparations Not to be used by persons with glaucoma or excessive pressure within the eye, by elderly persons (where undiagnosed glaucoma or excessive pressure within the eye may be present), or by children under 12 years of age, unless directed by a physician.

Sodium Perborate Mouthwash, Gargle, and Toothpaste Discontinue use if irritation or inflammation develops, or increases. Avoid swallowing.

Sulfur Preparation for External Use If undue skin irritation develops or increases, discontinue use and consult a physician.

Throat Preparations for Temporary Relief of Minor Sore Throat: Lozenges, Troches, Washes, Gargles, etc. Severe or persistent sore throat or sore throat accompanied by high fever, headache, nausea, and vomiting may be serious. Consult a physician promptly. Do not use more than 2 days or administer to children under 3 years of age unless directed by a physician.

Zinc Stearate Dusting Powders Keep out of the reach of infants and children; avoid inhaling.

INDEX

ABOUT THE AUTHORS

The authors have pooled their considerable experience in several important facets of the field of drugs in order to bring you the composite picture this book represents. Dr. Erwin Di Cyan has been a drug consultant for over 28 years, developing drugs for pharmaceutical companies for over-the-counter sale and prescription use. He is director of Di Cyan & Brown, drug consultants in New York, member of the American Chemical Society, New York Academy of Sciences, and other professional societies. Dr. Lawrence Hessman is a board-certified internist practicing internal medicine and gastroenterology. He is chief of internal medicine at Lowell General Hospital, Lowell, Massachusetts.